The Virtual Couch

This book is one of the first systematic examinations on the looming mental health crisis emerging from the COVID-19 pandemic from a psychoanalytic perspective.

Bringing together practising therapists from Asia and Europe, this book:

- analyses themes like anxiety, depression, sexuality, loss and death through clinical vignettes
- highlights how children, adolescents and adults have been responding to the pandemic
- explores how personal and collective trauma are mourned, remembered, repeated and worked through
- studies deep-seated prejudices and fears
- focuses on how the pandemic has stimulated exceptional manifestations of human solidarity and creativity

Comprehensive and practical, this book will be an essential guide for mental health professionals, counsellors, therapists and medical doctors treating psychological trauma.

Sonali Jain is Associate Professor of English in Bharati College, University of Delhi. Her doctoral work at Jawaharlal Nehru University (JNU) centred on Vijay Tendulkar and the semiotics of cinema. She was Translator-in-Residence at the University of East Anglia, UK, in 2008 and has translated Tendulkar's play *Baby* into English. She has also edited Strindberg's *Miss Julie*. She co-edited *Literature, Language, and the Classroom: Essays for Promodini Varma*, published by Routledge in 2021. Her areas of interest include psychoanalytic theory, film studies, drama and translation. She has been painting for many years, and her works have been exhibited in a number of group shows.

The Virtual Couch

COVID-19 through a
Psychoanalytic Lens

Edited by Sonali Jain

Routledge
Taylor & Francis Group

LONDON AND NEW YORK

Designed cover image: Painting by Sonali Jain.

First published 2023
by Routledge
4 Park Square, Milton Park, Abingdon, Oxon OX14 4RN

and by Routledge
605 Third Avenue, New York, NY 10158

Routledge is an imprint of the Taylor & Francis Group, an informa business

British Library Cataloguing-in-Publication Data
A catalogue record for this book is available from the British Library

Library of Congress Cataloging-in-Publication Data
A catalog record has been requested for this book

ISBN: 978-1-032-14060-5 (hbk)
ISBN: 978-1-032-18718-1 (pbk)
ISBN: 978-1-003-25589-5 (ebk)

DOI: 10.4324/9781003255895

Typeset in Sabon
by Apex CoVantage, LLC

This book is dedicated to the memory of my father
Surendra Singh Jain
who was delighted that I had taken up this project
but did not live to see it reach fruition.

Contents

Contributors

Sudhir Kakar is an eminent psychoanalyst and writer who lives in Goa, India. He is a major figure in the fields of cultural psychology and the psychology of religion. He has been listed as one of the world's 25 major thinkers as well as one of the 21 important thinkers of the twenty-first century.

Kakar was trained in psychoanalysis at the Sigmund-Freud Institute in Frankfurt, Germany. During 1976–1977, he was Professor and Head, Department of Humanities and Social Sciences at IIT Delhi. He has held visiting appointments and fellowships at the universities of Harvard, Chicago, McGill, Melbourne, Hawaii and Vienna, and INSEAD, France. He has been a Fellow at the Institute of Advanced Study, Princeton; Institute of Advanced Study, Berlin; Centre for Advanced Study of Humanities, University of Cologne. He is Honorary Professor, GITAM University, Visakhapatnam, as well as Visiting Professor, Goa University. His many honours include the Kardiner Award of Columbia University, Boyer Prize of the American Anthropological Association, Germany's Goethe Medal, Rockefeller Residency, McArthur Fellowship, Homi Bhabha Senior Fellowship, Merck-Tagore Award, Nehru and ICSSR National Fellowships and Distinguished Service Award of the Indo-American Psychiatric Association. He is a member of several academies around the world. In February 2012, he was conferred the Order of Merit of the Federal Republic of Germany, the country's highest civilian order.

Kakar is a prolific writer, with more than 25 books spanning a wide range of non-fiction as well as fiction. Four volumes of his collected essays are under preparation for publication by Oxford University Press in its series Great Thinkers of Modern Asia.

Nupur Dhingra Paiva is a chartered clinical psychologist, an associate fellow with the British Psychological Society, and a child psychotherapist. She started *Family Tree: Child and Adolescent Mental Health team* in New Delhi in 2018. She taught 'Infant Observation' as part of the Psychotherapy course at Ambedkar University Delhi from 2012 to 2020. She is also a certified Intensive Short-Term Dynamic Psychotherapy practitioner and trainer. Along with her husband, Richard Paiva, she is a co-founder of *The Art of Sport* – a development programme for girls, using sport and group therapy, based in New Delhi.

Shweta Dharamdasani is a trained psychoanalytic psychotherapist with an MPhil from Ambedkar University Delhi. She is also a rehabilitation psychologist certified by the Rehabilitation Council of India. She is a researcher and writer; her area of interest is in how culture and psyche influence each other. She is currently working with *Family Tree*, a mental health team for children and adolescents. She also facilitates a group of young girls at *The Art of Sport*.

Rekha Sapra is Officiating Principal of Bharati College, University of Delhi. Her work is in the area of psychology, women's empowerment and family welfare. She is the recipient of several awards: Jagmohan Krishna Das Award 2011, Meritorious Teacher Award by the Delhi Government 2013–2014 and Atal National Award 2019. She has authored five books and published research articles in international books and journals covering critical learnings and insights on parenting, social and emotional competence among children, resilience and coping among children during critical circumstances like COVID-19. She collaborates with many NGOs to promote the cause of early education and women's empowerment at the grassroots level. She has worked with schools in Delhi for children with attention-deficit hyperactivity disorder (ADHD).

Neetu Sarin is a psychologist and psychoanalyst at the Indian Psychoanalytical Society (IPS) and the International Psychoanalytical Association (IPA), London. Formerly, she taught at the School of Human Studies, Ambedkar University Delhi. Her expertise lies in bridging cultural and clinical realities, especially in areas of trauma. She serves on several international psychoanalytic committees, such as the Committee on Women and Psychoanalysis (COWAP-IPA), and the Cultural Outreach Committee (International Association of Relational Psychoanalysis and Psychotherapy). She works clinically with people suffering from psychosis, personality disorders and dissociative disorders. She was awarded the prestigious Sudhir Kakar Prize (2016) for best psychoanalytic writing under 40.

Ahmad Fuad Rahmat is Assistant Professor of Media and Digital Cultures at the University of Nottingham Malaysia. He is also a member of the Centre for Lacanian Analysis in New Zealand. He was trained in philosophy and cultural studies and has been published in journals such as *Radical Philosophy*, the *European Journal of Psychoanalysis* and *Psychoanalysis, Culture & Society*.

Jhuma Basak is a psychoanalyst based in Kolkata. She is a training and supervising analyst with the IPS. She is Co-Chair of Allied Centres of International New Groups (ING), IPA, London, and Member of the

IPA-IPSO Relations Committee. She is also a consultant to the COWAP-IPA. She is the founder of the Mira Centre for Innovation, Kolkata, which seeks to nurture a comprehensive environment of humanness. The philosophy followed encompasses the qualities of empathy, gratitude and compassion, while engaging with psychoanalysis, education and arts.

Namita Bhutani is a psychoanalytic psychotherapist currently in private practice in Delhi. She is a candidate with the IPS. She undertakes long-term work with adults. She has worked for the past 20 years in the field of mental health and has been associated with NGOs and hospitals in the field of disability, with children in need of care and protection and with women survivors of violence. She has also undertaken research work in these areas. Her interest lies in studying autistic states of withdrawal, melancholy, states of anxiety, regeneration of hope and movement through faith.

Rashi Kapoor is a training candidate in psychoanalysis with the Delhi chapter of the IPS, Kolkata, and the IPA, London. She works in private practice in New Delhi and is a consultant psychoanalytic psychotherapist with the Department of Mental Health and Behavioural Sciences at Fortis Healthcare, Delhi. She works with people in one-to-one psychotherapy and has a key interest in exploring issues at the cusp of feminism and psychoanalysis. Her current research interests focus on exploring the body as a site of processing psychic trauma.

Ashis Roy is a psychoanalytic therapist. He works with adults and couples. His interest is in clinical and cultural psychoanalysis. He was faculty at Ambedkar University Delhi and is presently faculty at CAPA. His book *Intimate Hindu-Muslim Relationships: A Psychoanalytic Exploration of the Self and the Other* will be published by SAGE-Yoda Press in 2023.

Gohar Homayounpour is a psychoanalyst and Gradiva Award–winning author. She is a member of the IPA and the American Psychoanalytic Association, a training and supervising psychoanalyst of the Freudian Group of Tehran and a scientific board member of the Freud Museum in Vienna. Her book *Persian Blues, Psychoanalysis and Mourning* was published by Routledge in August 2022.

Anne Gagnant de Weck is a former student of the Ecole Normale Supérieure in Lyon. She currently teaches in high schools and gives courses in university. In 2018, she defended a PhD in sociology dedicated to the contemporary practice of psychotherapies in Delhi. A book based on her doctoral work, titled *Un divan à Delhi. Psychothérapie et individualisme dans l'Inde contemporaine*, published by ENS Editions, will be released in May 2023 in France.

Benjamin Lévy is a former student of philosophy at the Ecole Normale Supérieure de Paris. He graduated in psychology from the Université Paris

Diderot and completed his doctoral thesis in 2016. Now a psychologist and psychoanalyst, he has published many papers and translations. He currently teaches introductory lessons in psychoanalysis at the Ecole des Psychologues Praticiens de Paris.

Surabhika Maheshwari is Associate Professor of Psychology at Indraprastha College for Women, University of Delhi, and a practising psychologist. With nearly two decades of experience, she is passionately involved in the teaching and practice of psychology. Her areas of interest include mental health, psychotherapy, psychology of identity and self. She has been an invited speaker at various prestigious platforms and has worked on projects with several organizations, including the World Health Organization (WHO). She has co-edited a special issue on Identity and Self of the Springer journal *Psychological Studies*.

Ananya Kushwaha is a psychoanalytic candidate with the IPS. She practises in Delhi as a part of a shared practice, The Psychotherapist Collective, with four other psychoanalytic candidates. She is also the director of a new non-profit initiative called Zeest – Centre for Psycho-Societal Innovation. Her clinical interests psychoanalytically have been in the areas of death and sexuality, masculinity, experiencing recognition as experiencing self, love and desire, analyst's desire and, most lately, democracy and psychoanalysis, divided subjectivity, narcissistic closure, feminine ethics and so on. Using the psychoanalytic method for developing community-based trainings and interventions is also her current preoccupation.

Urvashi Pawar is a psychoanalytical psychotherapist in New Delhi, India. She has been practising for the past 12 years and works primarily with adolescents, adults and couples. She completed her post-graduation from the Anna Freud Centre, UCL, London, in psychoanalytic developmental psychology after completing a post-graduation in clinical psychology from Delhi University. She is working at a private hospital in New Delhi and also has her private practice. She is a candidate with the IPA and the IPS.

Anurag Mishra is a psychiatrist and psychoanalytical psychotherapist trained in India and Europe. He is the Chief of the Psychoanalytical Unit at Fortis Healthcare, India. He is the founder of several organizations: Psychoanalysis India, which helped to organize the International Psychoanalytical Conferences and Sigmund Freud Talks in Delhi; Livonics Publishing, which has been publishing books on psychoanalysis and mental health, among others; Livonics Infotech and Livonics Institute of Integrated Learning and Research (www.liilr.livonics.com), which is engaged in interdisciplinary research and education. He currently resides in Latvia and is Academic Advisor to the University of Latvia International Institute of Indic Studies in Riga. He is the co-editor of *Psychoanalysis from the Indian Terroir*, along with Anup Dhar and Manasi Kumar.

Bhaskar Mukherjee is a psychiatrist based in Kolkata. His main areas of interest are treatment-resistant schizophrenia and treatment-resistant obsessive compulsive disorder. He is trained in molecular neuroscience, and is a psychiatrist as well as a practitioner of clinical molecular neuroscience. He sees psychiatric disorders from a lifetime perspective and does genetic counselling, orders molecular genetics testing if needed and educates patients about the real molecular neuroscientific basis of their diseases. His work has been published in *European Psychiatry* and other journals. He also serves as a resource person in various national and international psychiatric conferences.

Anup Dhar is a former professor of psychology and a former professor of philosophy. He has co-authored several books on globalization and capitalism, published by Routledge and other international publishers. His co-edited books include *Psychoanalysis from the Indian Terroir* (2018). He is currently working on an annotated edition of the English writings of the Indian psychoanalyst Girindrasekhar Bose. He is the editor of the *Journal of Practical Philosophy* and a member of the Editorial Board of *Rethinking Marxism*. He is currently teaching a two-year online course titled 'Psychoanalysis in Practice: Between Philosophy and Neurobiology'.

Foreword

The thoughtful and thought-provoking essays in this volume are a very welcome effort by psychoanalytic psychotherapists to turn the unique lens of psychoanalysis on issues around mental health that have come to the fore in the time of the COVID pandemic.

On a societal level, the pandemic is a singular event in that with both adults and children confined to home for long periods and socially isolated, normal lives have been radically upended. Psychologically, the pandemic has made the outside world seem dangerous and untrustworthy. There is a constant fear of catching the virus. Not only from strangers but also from friends and, even more unsettling, from parents, siblings, spouses and children, who normally constitute our unconscious envelope of safety, persons to whom we otherwise entrust our well-being without a thought. The virus itself is an uncanny object, all around us yet invisible, mounting further assault on our sense of what Erik Erikson called 'basic trust', the trust in the world being a benign place. This basic trust has its origins in the earliest years of life from an infant's experience of good-enough parenting that makes the outer world, at the time essentially consisting of the family, safe and predictable. With a decrease in basic trust and the wilting of the plant that grows out of its soil, hope, our collective psychic economy is in doldrums. The signs, a marked increase in anxiety disorders, substance abuse, messy separations of couples, to mention only a few of the mental health issues, are everywhere.

The increase in death by suicide is the most clear-cut expression of a widespread decrease in basic trust and hopefulness. Besides the fear of being infected and thus becoming a social pariah, there are the threats of financial ruin, looming joblessness and social isolation that increase the risk of suicide in vulnerable populations. Suicide itself, the act of snuffing out one's own life, is characterized by a complete loss of hope. The final curtain descending on the mind of a person who commits suicide is of hopelessness, the stage going utterly dark with the loss of all hope. To someone with already existing mental health issues whose balance between trust and mistrust was always precarious, the hope always feeble, the pandemic can give the final push into hopelessness and thus into suicide.

To varying degrees, the general decrease of basic trust has also spilt over to the society's institutions, especially of the government but also the media, politics, medicine and education. In part, the hesitancy or refusal to be vaccinated reflects the decrease of trust in the institutions of the state entrusted with this task. Has there been any social institution that has been a beneficiary of the pandemic? I would answer this question in the affirmative and say, yes, the family, the earliest source of safety in an unpredictable world even if did not completely escape the mistrust created by the pandemic. For it is the family where the existential question of 'Can I trust the world?' was once answered with a resounding 'Yes'.

With the ending of the pandemic, basic trust in the outside world, which varies in individuals depending on their experience within the family during infancy, will not be automatically reinstated. For some time, even with the restoration of social and economic forces that were inimical to the traditional family, the family will continue to benefit from the trust-surplus generated by the pandemic, a surplus that will also trickle down to the larger community in which the family is embedded.

The editor is to be congratulated for bringing together psychoanalytic therapists from different countries to reflect upon a contemporary issue of signal import that continues to preoccupy people all over the world. In doing so, she has also countered a widespread perception that psychoanalysts have no interest in or respect for reality.

Sudhir Kakar

Acknowledgements

I thank Professor Sudhir Kakar for being generous enough to find the time to write the Foreword to this volume. His insights are unparalleled and have helped sharpen the focus of this book. Thank you, Sir.

I am also sincerely grateful to Dr Anurag Mishra. This volume would not have been possible without your encouragement and contribution. I must add that your sense of humour kept me afloat.

I thank all contributors, whose experiences and insights have helped shape this book. I must make special mention of Dr Mamta Shah: thank you for quieting my anxiety and doubts and always giving me a patient ear.

I extend my thanks to Dr Promodini Varma for her sure, steady succour and her unconditional help. I am grateful to Dr Rekha Sapra, Principal Bharati College, whose interest and encouragement go beyond her chapter. I also thank other colleagues at Bharati College, especially Preeti and Bhawna, who gave timely technical help.

I am indebted to my mother and to my sisters Sushmita and Surbhi for their unconditional love and care, and to all friends who stood by me and mitigated my blues.

Thank you Amitabha and Pinky for containing me. Thank you for your warm support and cheer.

Introduction

Sonali Jain

Do you wonder where we have gone?
Multitudes
Painless?
Caught unawares without our last breath!
Nostrils stuffed.
We ceased to be human
And could not pause . . .
Time relentless. Perhaps too kind.
No more.
Why blame the virus?
We're off the brink
'Dying our own death.'

The Yaksha asked: 'What is the greatest wonder in the world?' Yudhishthira replied: 'Every day, men see creatures depart to Yama's abode and yet, those who remain seek to live forever. This verily is the greatest wonder.'
(*Mahabharata*, trans. C. Rajagopalachari, 1974, p. 142)

The COVID-19 pandemic has thrown up unprecedented challenges to life and to sanity. It has seared through social, psychological, economic and cultural contexts, almost taking us back in time. Since March 2020, the pendulum of responses to the pandemic has swung both ways. On the one hand, it swept us through the tough journey of anxiety, loss, death and bereavement. On the other, one cannot but concede that for many it has been a time for reflection, and some perhaps struck upon new facets of themselves, becoming productive and prolific with online work. Many others found their own corner, becoming inspired and creative; many others found a good space in solitude, becoming pensive yet engaged.

Bereavement is an extremely painful and consuming experience. Anxiety disorder and major depression may follow. Loss of family, loved ones, dear friends – the suddenness with which COVID-positive cases embraced death during the pandemic was alarming. There was not even time for proper

DOI: 10.4324/9781003255895-1

mourning. The dread of death, as Becker has pointed out, lies at the core of the experience of being human (Becker, 1973). We have the ability to anticipate and reflect on our own death, and so we live our lives 'forever shadowed by the knowledge that we will grow, blossom, and inevitably, diminish and die' (Yalom, 2008, p. 1). As the playwright Samuel Beckett has said, 'They give birth astride of a grave, the light gleams an instant, then it's night once more' (Beckett, 1959, p. 89).

To escape the terror of death, people also took recourse to religion, to nationalist sentiment, joining groups so that they would not feel isolated. Even as 'social distancing' became the need of the hour, attachment and proximity to loved ones was what was desired. However, paradoxically, social distancing won out. We insulated ourselves, with books, music, games, newspapers, anything we could bury ourselves in, to distance ourselves emotionally from this chilling reality.

The pandemic has stimulated exceptional manifestations of human solidarity and creativity, for which there must be gratitude, though it has also brought to the fore some of our most deep-seated fears and prejudices. It would also be relevant to explore health as one end of the spectrum, especially the turn to forms of traditional healing. Sudhir Kakar discusses this in good detail in his book *Shamans, Mystics and Doctors* (Kakar, 1991).

Psychoanalysts have been struggling to come to grips with a host of issues that have arisen in these simmering times. On the one hand, while the real psychoanalytic couch has lain vacant, on the other, analysts have been inundated with therapy sessions. The loss of the real couch, and its replacement by a virtual one, is experienced as deprivation by both the analysand and the analyst.

The virtual world

In this section, I address the central question: What do we mean by the *virtual couch*? I have applied this term to various online platforms like Skype and Zoom, which are being employed to carry on psychoanalysis. Adjusting to phone sessions can be extremely time-consuming for the analyst and the analysand. The analysand may find high levels of anxiety stirring up, especially around the quiet, even the silences and speech in a virtual session. He or she may experience feelings of not receiving the gentle and benevolent maternal, possibly not receiving a good-enough space for alliance.

Important questions arise: how does one express empathy on the virtual couch? Is it resilience on the part of the analyst and of the analysand that keeps psychoanalytic work going? In this virtual reality, online platforms are being used, which poses a challenge to both analysand and analyst. Both analyst and analysand also seem to have a choice: both may choose to not see each other in an audio session or see each other on a virtual platform, something which happened only occasionally earlier. Body language may be fully or partially invisible depending on the mode of the online session.

Hickey et al. (2021) have reviewed the available literature on the impact of technology on transference and countertransference both before and during the pandemic. They note that in classical psychoanalysis, there is a tradition of maintaining the analyst's privacy and neutrality, and self-disclosure is used sparingly, if at all. Due to the absence of the analysts' online presence, analysands may seek to re-create them on a virtual level by online searching. The analyst often is unaware of the important material that may be unearthed or re-created by the analysand through online means and, therefore, does not have the opportunity to work through such material. The possibility of such online searches by the analysand, which compromise the tradition of the therapist's privacy, of course, already existed before COVID-19, but the pandemic exacerbated the tendency. Patients may construct extensive fantasies about their therapists based on what they find online. Such material can be a rich source of transferential feelings which can lead to important unconscious meanings and discoveries.

Susan Pacey (2021) points out that the pandemic tests both analysand and analyst in similar ways. Indeed, analysts also have their own need for a connection with others, which may get aggravated in the face of a continuous mortal threat. Pacey asks, 'How then in this crisis do practitioners sustain themselves enough to be able to engage with and contain their clients' anxieties?'

Sigmund Freud maintained that 'anxiety in children is originally nothing other than an expression of the fact that they are feeling the loss of the person they love' (Freud, 1905/1953, p. 224). In a later essay, he wrote: 'anxiety appears as the reaction to the felt loss of the object' (Freud, 1926/1959, p. 137). Anxiety is determined also by the threat of losing the love of the object. Freud also distinguished between anxiety as a reaction to the danger of loss and the pain of mourning, which is a reaction to the actual loss of the object (Freud, 1926/1959).

A psychoanalytic perspective recognizes that there is an inability to contain loss personally as well as socially and culturally, throwing up defences: denial and displacement as also the 'paranoid elaboration of mourning' (Fornari, 1975, p. xviii). This perspective looks at how personal and collective trauma are mourned, remembered, repeated and worked through.

Psychoanalysts have reflected on the issue of temporality, which is also at the heart of psychoanalysis, and how time has been transformed. Dana Birksted-Breen (2021) says: 'The new experience of remote sessions has created the possibility of "unpicking" the threads of the usual setting, enabling authors to develop ideas about what is normally left silent.' Thus, one of the aims of this volume is also to understand and examine, with a psychoanalytic lens, the ways in which time has been transformed during the COVID-19 pandemic.

Though technically there may not be any difference in the transaction between analysand and analyst regarding payment of fee, in psychoanalysis money has been considered 'emotional currency', to use Anca Carrington's term. With difficulties around money shooting up, many analysands could be dropping out of analysis because their own earnings and savings are getting depleted. However, analysts cannot keep reducing their fee because money is a significant boundary in psychoanalysis: 'Money has not so much of a role in the external world, but in an internal economy ruled by phantasy and whose foundations are as old as the beginning of the psyche itself' (Carrington, 2015, p. xiv). Analysands leaving therapy because of lack of money and an inability to pay for sessions can be experienced by analysts in different ways.

Education has faced a plethora of changes and challenges in the face of the corona crisis. As I write this, I have just got back to facing my students after almost two years. The connect between teacher and student, the holding environment, to use Winnicott's (1960) formulation, has been missing. Online teaching, which basically boils down to speaking and listening, often without a face and usually without a question, paves the way for boredom to set in. The microphone at one end, the laptop at the other, is an utterly unlikely substitute for the physical space of the classroom and the physical presence of students and teachers. Both teaching and testing have got a severe jolt as we grapple with the effects of the pandemic on education at all levels, from primary school to higher educational institutions.

In this book

All chapters in this book are a response to the pandemic and the ways in which it has affected our lives: ways in which children, adolescents and adults have responded in their inner and outer worlds to complex emotions. Anxiety, depression, sexuality, loss, death and suicide due to the pandemic are some responses that are dwelt upon.

As Sudhir Kakar points out in the Foreword, basic trust has its origins in the earliest years of life. It is an infant's experience of good-enough parenting that makes the outer world, at the time essentially consisting of the family, safe and predictable. With a decrease in basic trust and the wilting of the plant that grows out of its soil, hope, our collective psychic economy is in the doldrums.

Nupur Dhingra Paiva and Shweta Dharamdasani, in their chapter, have pointed out some striking and poignant examples of children and adolescents affected by various phases of the lockdown. In the initial weeks of the lockdown when many, who had no safe homes in the cities, were leaving in hordes along with their children, the media insensitively referred to them as 'migrant workers', 'a label that conveniently prioritised the economic and took the human out of the narrative'. They add that 'in a parallel universe of those people who were privileged enough to retain their homes and screens to disappear into, we again forgot about the children', making them largely invisible. Or wishing they would be. The chapter contains several interesting vignettes of children's play during the pandemic, which illustrate how children have been coping with a situation where school and friends are missing. Play became all indoors, dependent only on the objects available in the home as well as upon the child's imagination.

Rekha Sapra uses the notion of the inner child – a direct representation of oneself in early developmental years. The inner child holds memories, emotions as well as good and bad experiences. The negative and harmful words and actions of caregivers make the child feel threatened and unsafe. The wounded inner child influences and moulds the adult personality, exercising immense power over the relationships and decisions of the adult. The response of adults with a wounded inner child to the pandemic needs to be investigated in order to assess the long-term consequences of home quarantine for an extended duration.

Neetu Sarin, commenting upon the 'turning inwards' necessitated by the pandemic as a 'powerful antidote to the manic productivity of society', distinguishes between this 'turning inwards' and the more severe form of detachment, called 'psychic withdrawal'. She elaborates on Meltzer's idea of dimensionality and notes the limitation of the two-dimensional virtual world: 'the more we rely on screens to keep us alive, the more depleted we become in imagination'. Dreaming, she proposes, may be used as a thread that ties together the fragmented parts of ourselves in these times.

Ahmad Fuad Rahmat focuses upon the relevance of psychoanalysis for a COVID world by revisiting Lacan's account of analysts as witnesses to the unconscious. According to him, the significance of the failure of knowledge is essential. It is at the failure of knowledge that the unconscious's uncertain and fluid quality may be captured. The author asserts: 'The general outline of the Lacanian approach . . . has the advantage of grounding psychoanalytic work in crisis mode.' Modernity, according to Lacan, is a series of traumas that constantly 'reveals the tenuousness of our symbolic resources'. The COVID crisis is just another in a series of crises, which highlights the urgent need for analysis.

Jhuma Basak, referencing Michael Eigen, asserts a loneliness common and basic to all natures. Eigen makes a clear distinction between loneliness and solitude. All, even children, can well internalize the human predicament at a critical, traumatic locale – particularly as witnessed in the COVID-19 situation, faced, as we all were, with a harrowing time of death and devastation. Basak posits that mentalization becomes a unique converging point of thought, reflection, symbolization and containment of affect. She argues that the ego may be integrated with the external world and its objects as she intertwines Japanese cultural, social and psychological contexts into her arguments. Basak makes mention of street life a good deal as she writes about the impact of natural disasters and focuses on the COVID distress which has ravaged community life.

Namita Bhutani writes about how this time of limited movement and space has resonated differently with different people. She draws on Donald Meltzer's concept of dimensionality as well as the recent work of Alina

Schellekes on arid mental landscapes. Using a series of clinical vignettes, she illustrates how a state of mental and emotional lockdown can arise from different parts: 'a desire to not acknowledge reality, a difficulty or refusal to process what is going on inside and outside, a wish to minimize pain, a giving up of hope and agency'.

Rashi Kapoor's chapter aims at assessing and enunciating the extent of psychological distress that the pandemic has inflicted on our notions of closeness and intimacy. Even the most intimate cannot touch another, no matter how close. Using the analogy of a patient infected with genital herpes (HSV-2), Kapoor notes how carrying the virus loads the carrier with a responsibility: that of a huge possibility of infecting another. She discusses how the terror of that responsibility translates into the stigma that is carried by the infected. Wondering if the infected person is no more than the infection, and if it wipes out everything else that makes a person an individual, she argues that illnesses reveal something deep inside of us, our own histories as well as our transgenerational histories.

Ashis Roy suggests that the number of deaths and the suddenness with which the pandemic has completely ravaged the self and surroundings requires a newer way of thinking about mourning and loss within the psyche. Based on his clinical work in a university setting, he reflects on the suffering of young people as they are unable to feel integrated within themselves. Ignorance about mental health issues, he asserts, 'can lead to a false sense that each individual is born with the capacity to deal with the possibility of death to others and to oneself'.

Gohar Homayounpour attempts to take a look at the paradox of the COVID-19 pandemic in the particular socio-political situation in Iran and observes how it has led to an attack on intimacy while accentuating the feelings of fear and loss. Iran had to deal with the outbreak while simultaneously having to deal with an ongoing economic crisis that has lasted for decades. Homayounpour posits that her patients find solidarity and solace in this oft-repeated assertion: 'At least we are not in this alone.' In being able to establish this link with the outside world, there is a sense of solidarity. This is a fresh perspective which needs to be acknowledged and to be accepted with some gratitude in fact.

Anne Gagnant de Weck and Benjamin Lévy give us a fascinating view of the pandemic as seen by analysts in France, based on in-depth interviews with 18 psychoanalysts carried out through Zoom by film directors Clovis Stocchetti and Pascal Laethier, the latter also a psychoanalyst. Gagnant and Lévy have also carried out a survey of the relevant literature. They find that French therapists fall into three broad groups. The first – a small minority – consists of those who refused to follow up by any electronic means. The second group comprises those who were already used to online work with their patients and for whom the pandemic did not pose too big a challenge. In between these extremes come the majority, who reluctantly adopted whatever electronic means they could find to continue their work with patients.

Surabhika Maheshwari, in her chapter 'The Waves of Loss', states that grief is a complex emotion that can be experienced and expressed in a variety of ways, depending upon each person's individual circumstances. She also argues that we must learn to distinguish between grief and loss as well as understand the different shades of each. While enumerating the different types of griefs that can be experienced, she points out that one must also understand the different stages of the emotion and that very often mourning can begin much before the actual loss occurs. The pandemic exacerbated the feelings of helplessness and desolation that grief brings in its wake, and much work will be required to overcome its effects.

Shweta Dharamdasani examines the terms *trauma* and *loss* from a psychoanalytic angle. She begins her exploration with her own response to the news of the death of two celebrities and her memories of her deceased grandfather, as they fall on a common day. The news made her wonder about the process of mourning in the absence of rituals due to the restrictions imposed during the pandemic. The second aperture is the collective response at a societal level, while the third is through a clinical vignette.

Ananya Kushwaha writes that the pandemic has highlighted and exaggerated our existing mental lockdown and isolation, our 'distancing' from 'contact' of any kind through its imperative of 'bodily distancing'. Kushwaha claims how, in India, overlapping with the spirit of the times, a cultural shift has taken place in the direction of focus on the 'self' and on freedom for its discovery and its expression. She claims that most psychoanalytical therapists and psychologists in general will affirm that the referrals they have received have significantly increased over this last decade or so. The bulk of the chapter consists of interviews with common people carried out by the author's colleagues. These capture the helplessness experienced by people due to dislocation and loss of livelihood while also containing stories of coping and solidarity.

Urvashi Pawar, in her provocatively titled chapter 'Unmasked: The Dread of Being Able to Kill', focuses on one significant aspect of the impact of the pandemic among people: the capacity of infecting another person, and living with the feeling that we caused someone to die. She points out that we are all under the threat of the virus, which can attack us in insidious ways; the unknown plagues therapists and patients alike. It isn't 'safe-enough' for the patient and the therapist to meet each other. Work goes on in physically distanced modes. She notes that it is memories of their violent and murderous wishes that have become available to the patients. In analysis we often face our aggressive wishes and internal attacks, and the coronavirus has made us fear our internalized enraged attacks and destructive phantasies turning into reality. Phantasies that had been repressed erupt volcanically, and patients are enveloped in this storm of annihilation anxiety, separation anxiety and guilt of destructive wishes, among many other unthinkable anxieties.

Last but not the least: where are our brains? The question is rhetorical, posing to the reader: where are your brains? The book closes with a trialogue. Three doyens of psychiatry and philosophy are in animated conversation with one another. As one encounters new words and novel theories that they bring up, complementing one another, the process becomes rich for the audience. Focusing on the problem of 'brain', the tripartite dialogue among Anurag Mishra, Bhaskar Mukherjee and Anup Dhar – which happened between the second and the third wave of the COVID-19 pandemic – examines in a 'disruptive and integrative' manner the intertwined foldings of the neuronal, the linguistic and the affective bodies. In the larger sphere of 'mental health', new questions arose during the pandemic, such as what lockdown, quarantine and social distancing could do to the human species. The question is not whether psychotherapy or psychoanalysis will be or can be conducted online; important as it is, it is a question of just the 'setting'. The more important question is: 'how do we make sense of the human and the non-human brain-mind complex in the twenty-first century; what kind of new philosophical, scientific and socio-cultural question is the pandemic throwing up?' This chapter is an effort by all three not to clinch one position in favour of the other but to dialogue with patience, with care and so on.

Conclusion

COVID-19 has challenged the ways in which we, as a society, have been conducting ourselves. As we realize, the contributors to this volume are all practitioners, in different kinds of settings, in India and elsewhere, who have been dealing sensitively with people in mental distress during the pandemic. Their empathy, trust and sensitivity are evident from their writing. They have gone beyond chronicling their experiences and have raised issues and concerns regarding not only psychotherapy but how we, as human beings, interact with one another. I close with a poem:

> *In my dream I was far away*
> *Wishing to turn back and look at you –*
> *No luck, no chance.*
> *I cannot wait for you to die;*
> *My fire will extinguish with the roar of the unjust earth.*
> *An encounter, unexpected,*
> *Will fill us with terrible longing.*
> *The pendulum swings incessantly,*
> *An empty quietude, nothing to say.*
> *We apologise with our minds*
> *And gaze at the furnace without breath.*
> *No prayers after the inevitable.*
> *On our palette there's grey and white*
> *Held by death and despair.*

References

Becker, E. (1973). *The denial of death*. Simon & Schuster.

Beckett, S. (1959). *Waiting for Godot*. Faber & Faber.

Birksted-Breen, D. (2021). Editorial. *The International Journal of Psychoanalysis, 102*(1), 1–2. https://doi.org/10.1080/00207578.2021.1876318

Carrington, A. (Ed.). (2015). *Money as emotional currency*. Routledge.

Fornari, F. (1975). *The psychoanalysis of war*. Anchor-Doubleday Books.

Freud, S. (1953). Three essays on the theory of sexuality. In J. Strachey (Ed. & Trans.), *The standard edition of the complete psychological works of Sigmund Freud* (Vol. 7, pp. 125–243). Hogarth Press. (Original work published 1905)

Freud, S. (1959). Inhibitions, symptoms and anxiety. In J. Strachey (Ed. & Trans.), *The standard edition of the complete psychological works of Sigmund Freud* (Vol. 20, pp. 75–172). Hogarth Press. (Original work published 1926)

Hickey, C., Schubmehl, J. Q., & Beeber, A. (2021). Technology, transference, and COVID-19 – With reference to Davanloo's Intensive short-term dynamic psychotherapy. *British Journal of Psychotherapy, 38*(1), 116–135. https://doi.org/10.1111/bjp.12693

Kakar, S. (1991). *Shamans, mystics and doctors: A psychological inquiry into india and its healing traditions*. The University of Chicago Press.

Pacey, S. (2021). Thoughts on reading 'Aftershocks', a contemporary poem by A. E. Stallings. *Couple and Family Psychoanalysis, 11*, 216–218.

Rajagopalachari, C. (Trans.). (1974). *Mahabharata*. Bharatiya Vidya Bhavan.

Winnicott, D. W. (1960). The theory of the parent-child relationship. *The International Journal of Psychoanalysis, 41*, 585–595.

Yalom, I. D. (2008). *Staring at the sun: Overcoming the terror of death*. Josey-Bass.

1 Play

Seeing children's inner worlds

Nupur Dhingra Paiva and
Shweta Dharamdasani

#1

Four-year-old Jay installed a lockdown in his house with anything and everything that he could lay his hand on. As the world outside came to a standstill with the countrywide lockdown, the world inside Jay had a lot going on. Following is the description of his play by his mother.[1]

> Our four-year-old has been busy
> With Lockdown Installation Art.
> He creates lockdowns in the living room
> In the bedroom another
> And a third one in our front yard.
>
> Things are placed upside down
> Any exposed areas he wants to protect
> Are painstakingly covered in cardboard from pre-Corona days.
> Cushions, hammers, balance bikes and scooters
> Car jacks and slabs of wood
> In intricately inert inextricable togetherness
> Trapped and stuck to each other.
> These objects won't infect each other,
> He seems to say.
>
> All things have been catatonically compelled
> To stay in place and prevent passage
> Put there with artistic indolence.
> And with stubborn somnambulance
> Things stay unmoved. Through the day,
> We keep bumping into this stillness
> As I move through our lockdown space
> Emotion is stirred in me
> As if to make up for the
> Entrapment everywhere else.

DOI: 10.4324/9781003255895-2

#2

Eight-year-old Devina's imaginary play offers a view into the workings of the mind of a child stuck inside the house during the lockdown. Here is the description of her play during the early days into the lockdown, as described by her mother.

Devina set up a bus station. The foot mat was turned into a bus. The bus was moved around by dragging the mat by her feet. The schedule of arrival of buses was erratic. Sometimes they would come and sometimes they would not.

The mother (as a passenger) is told to wait for the bus. Meanwhile the bus has broken down. It has run out of gas. Devina, the driver, goes to ask for fuel. Her own shadow is the person she is asking help from. After some time, grudgingly she is given the help, and with some fuel, she is able to restart the bus.

Meanwhile, the stranded worker passenger (mother), who had no food or water with her, receives a call from the president, who wants flowers. She must deliver the flowers by 5 a.m. However, she has to wait for the bus to arrive.

The bus finally arrives with some food and water, and the stranded worker/passenger is (as instructed by Devina, the director of the play) shocked as it is an old rickety bus and not a new one. As it is an old bus, the worker/passenger has to push the bus. After all the difficulties and troubles, they finally reach the worker's/passenger's destination. And both the driver and the passenger start dancing in celebration.

#3

Nine-year-old Aarti was seen in therapy due to issues related to her feeling of anger, which would present itself as over-eating and issues related to control and expulsion of pent-up energy. The work in the initial days was online due to the lockdown. She would like to talk a lot and would experience sessions as shorter than what they were, always asking for more time, wishing she had three hours instead of one.

Aarti's play during the lockdown through the screen was all about building or drawing castles. During many of the sessions, she created her own fort. She was the princess of this fort. The fort was made by using chairs, bed sheets and blankets. The chairs were the pillars. The blue bed sheet became the roof as a sky and the green blanket provided cushioning for the floor to sit on. All her soft toys become characters that live with Princess Aarti in the fort. And she brought one of her favourite books to read: 'The girl who made no mistakes'. She liked to talk to the therapist from the fort as that made her feel comfortable and safe.

***

March 2020 did many things for India. One of those was to make our children invisible: make them disappear.[2]

For the initial weeks of the lockdown, the focus was on the horror of people leaving the cities in droves, along with their children. To the media, they were 'migrant workers' – a label that conveniently prioritized the economic and took the human out of the narrative. The fact that these were families leaving together was rarely focused on, but those were the stories that were drilled into our awareness at the time – Danish Siddiqui's photograph of the man walking with his child on his shoulders; the man who said he was lucky to have a cycle cart so he could put his children and meagre belongings on it because he had no work and no money to live in Delhi anymore; children who were walking along with their parents, having been uprooted from what was familiar, from schools and local *gullis*, headed to uncertainty. The photographs of small children straggling behind their parents or straddling their shoulders were heart-piercing but not enough to make these children count, it seemed. After the television-owning world in India watched the toddler trying to wake his dead mother on the railway platform, dead from starvation and misery, mainstream media did not keep up with that child (or for that matter, even the story). Mainstream media have not kept up with these children to find out what happened to them. They have all but disappeared from view.

In a parallel universe of those people who were privileged enough to retain their homes and screens to disappear into, we again forgot about the children. Apart from addressing the question of how not to interrupt the school curriculum, and hence, how to keep them occupied, we again made large parts of our children invisible. Or wished they would be. For over 18 months, the school corridors and playgrounds have been deserted, the after-school activity schedule has been blank and celebrations quiet. Have we paused to wonder where all that energy went? The energy that fuels daily learning, play, sport, competition, laughter, friendships, bullying, fist-fights and arguments with peers – it is not just lying dormant but is actively eating away at our children from the inside, killing their motivation and aspirations, a phenomenon which is loosely being referred to as 'mental health problems'. That is the more compassionate term. In many adult circles it is also being referred to as 'unmotivated', 'disinterested' and 'lazy'.

As a society, in 2020–2021 we have repeatedly proved that we largely see our people as compliant capital. We are interested in what resource they will provide, without asking complex or inconvenient questions; ergo, the young need to be made pliable just as the workers need to work. In doing so, as policy makers and educators, certainly as politicians and sometimes even as parents, we forget that we live our lives from the inside. When we make our children's internal worlds invisible, we do so at our own peril because this will return to cost all society, all communities, in the form of aggression both outward and turned inward as rising hatred, violent and petty crime, as well as suicide (Paiva, 2020).

* * *

Children need to play. Nowadays parents are all consumed with their children developing motor and cognitive skills through play, but our pitch here is different. Children need to play to make sense of their internal world and external worlds. For children, play is not just recreation or leisure, which implies that it is an indulgence, but important and serious work. It is pleasurable and engrossing precisely because it is emotional. Otherwise, it would merely be handling of the objects (Erikson, 1950; Paiva, 2018).

What speech/language does for adults, play does for children. Rather, sometimes the act of play does what even speech/language fails to do. With the sudden lockdown and shutting of all means of social interaction for children, it becomes important that the child plays. A child who is able to play it out is probably coping better than the one who is not (Erikson, 1950).

In nondirective approaches to play, all play is therapy. The child chooses to construct his or her play in a way that will best communicate to the adult/therapist his or her experience. The toys in a playroom serve as the instruments for metaphorical construction, which symbolizes internal, unnameable, emotional states.

If one wishes to understand a child, one needs to understand his or her play because it is through play that children express themselves, conveying what they cannot express in words. What a child chooses to play betrays 'his inner processes, desires, problems and anxieties' (Bettelheim, 1987). It is how children make sense of difficult feelings. Jealousy, anger, guilt and hatred are enacted between dolls and monsters – which makes it easier to handle them in real relationships. In play, the little child can escape from the impact of a situation that is too painful for him or her to accept as it stands. The child can escape for a little while by pretending that he or she is someone else.

For example, for 4-year-old Jay, his lockdown art installation allowed him to make some sense of the difficult reality and perhaps even have some sense of control. He placed large objects according to him and they could continue to stay as long as he wanted. In his play, objects could be kept together without the fear of infection. The installation allowed him to work through distress caused by distance both emotional and physical.

For 8-year-old Devina, play is serious business; her imaginary play is quite detailed and complex. Her play is a reflection of the real world outside. There is uncertainty and not-knowing that her play demonstrates. Devina in the play has taken up the role of the one who knows and who has much more charge of what happens. She projects herself as a capable person who can go and ask for fuel and is able to help the stranded worker reach her destination. The role reversal allows her to feel in power, the power to give instructions rather than to take instructions. It also captures the lack of resources that the stranded worker has in order to reach her destination. However, for Devina her play acts as a bridge to the acceptance of reality by enabling the feeling to be expressed and seen from different points of view, in a controlled way. The play has become a means to master this crisis and to feel competent and in control.

Aarti, in her rigorous, repetitive exertion of building the fort and creating a comforting and safe environment, expresses the need to feel comforted and safe. The communication can be about both physical and emotional safety. She feels safe in being able to sit in her fort, her space, with every soft toy of hers symbolically representing the support and cushioning that she needs in order to deal with feelings coming up at being stuck at home, towards her parents and other family members. In her space, she continues to be the girl who makes no mistakes, the mistake of letting her feelings out of her fort. Her drawings showed the defence of reaction formation at work. The treasure that was there in the castle was guarded by guards. One can safely say that the treasure here represents her feelings. Her feelings have to be guarded, and not only that, they have to be covered by hearts and stars. Since the expression of difficult and unpleasant feelings creates anxiety in her mother, they all have to be covered under everything that is starry and lovely.

* * *

The period 2020–2021 has been revealing. It has revealed so much of what lay hidden under the cover of productive activity, workplace objectives, targets and competition. The emotional world has made its presence felt.[3]

Pre-COVID, our small-but-effective child and adolescent mental health team in New Delhi had a steady trickle of one new referral a week. Over the past months that has turned into a deluge, representing the increasing levels of anguish in families, led by the children, ensuring that our team had to return to work face to face, because emotional distress does not engage too well over a digital medium. In many cases, the tides of children's emotional lives had numerous outlets in 'normal' times, and parents could get by thinking of them as merely niggling worries: the occasional scratch the child inflicted on themselves, the occasional nightmare or the occasional sibling squabble. These could no longer be ignored when everyone was together at home for months. Strained relationships could no longer be avoided, resentments and rivalries could no longer be hidden, and 'teenage angst' could no longer be a dismissive depiction. After all, we are in lockdown with our feelings.

There is a pattern to the forms of distress we are seeing: a 6-year-old fears earthquakes and is constantly anxious, unwilling to let a parent out of sight. A 9-year-old is afraid of death, troubled by events in other parts of the world where people have been killed. A 12-year-old fears losing loved ones; another is preoccupied with her appearance, smoothening her hair many times a day, scrutinizing her face for blemishes. Many moody, quiet, reclusive 13-year-olds are spending hours on a screen, their world reduced to 13 inches, supposedly at school but navigating to websites far-far-away. The boys' locker room incident that received so much public attention in the summer of 2020 could also be seen as an example of young people's sexuality and aggression emerging – through misogynistic, hateful talk. Hyperactive, angry children, unable to hear 'no', unable to sit still. Others who are smoking cannabis and using alcohol or pornographic material and gaming to tranquilise themselves (Paiva, 2022).

We don't all experience or process distress in the same way. There are differences in how our children's distress shows up depending on their age, temperament, developmental life stage and previous history. In many cases we find that the current situation only exacerbated or unearthed an existing problem that the family was papering over. It would be foolishness to believe that 'the kids are alright'.

A 7-year-old boy was brought in by his parents saying he was being explosive. He was experiencing immense rage towards a loved aunt who was leaving to go back to her country of residence after the lockdown lifted, but underneath that explosion was a massive fear of losing her and fear that she won't come back. This fear of loss was pushing out as explosions where he would shout, cry and throw things.

In many cases where parents are now working from home, the lines between office hours and family time have blurred. Activities like reading, which was an integral part of bedtime routine pre-COVID, have fizzled out for 10-year-old Rahul, for instance, since everyone is at home and 'spending time' together all the time. As far as Rahul is concerned, he has less quality time now with his parents. This makes him angry with them and brings on anxiety. The acknowledgement of loss without masking it under 'we could have had it worse', along with resumption of the bedtime routine of reading, pillow fights and honest conversations around who misses what parts of their lives pre-pandemic, has subsequently helped relieve Rahul's symptoms of screaming and crying.

For 6-year-old Ketan, on the other hand, the initial phases of lockdown proved to be a relief for some time, wherein anxiety symptoms disappeared because now he knew he had his parents at home and they kept him close. This changed, however, as the world opened up somewhat in winter 2020 and his symptoms returned with greater intensity, coupled with the fear of loss and death.

Fifteen-year-old Smriti was struggling to deal with the loss of school/peer relationships/post-school activities and being forced to be privy to familial dynamics. The change in situation came as a shock to her, almost as though she was getting to know her parents up close for the first time. Her parents too were meeting this adolescent rebellious teenager after years; it was as though they had skipped seeing the progression towards adolescence in their child because external forces such as work commitments, schoolwork and after-school activities had kept them busy.

Seven-year-old Mili's fears latched onto something concrete and identifiable: a monster she stumbled upon on YouTube. This made her afraid of the dark, and so she ended up sleeping between her parents. She had experienced a series of losses during the pandemic – first her nanny had left abruptly to look after another child. Then Mili's best friend of six years changed neighbourhoods. From Mili's perspective, the people she loved kept leaving. Her fear of the dark and ending up in her parent's bed was a great solution to the original problem of loss; now she could keep an eye on her parents and prevent them from also disappearing.

What we are seeing in the clinic is representative of what is happening in some measure in every family, in every socio-economic stratum, in every community – with greater or lesser intensity. Not even a miniscule percentage of that gets attended to. We are sitting on a colossal time bomb of emotional distress that will blow up in our faces: anxiety, depression, aggression and self-sabotage, perhaps even suicide (NCRB, 2019; Rampal, 2020), will be the main symptoms.

***

Children under the age of five are designed to be close to family members and have active fantasy lives, seen through imaginative play. Attachment bonds are formed and strengthened by this age and form the bedrock for all future relationships. At this stage, social communication capacities are being built in small safe interactions with others who have been vetted by their carers. They are happy building tents under tables and talking to their dolls or dinosaurs. This is the easiest age group to manage at home with core attachment figures and without the social interaction that schools and playgrounds provide. Social skills cannot be learnt in isolation, though, so how these children learn to interact with other children will remain to be seen. Their distress is easier to soothe by providing the safety of family and the familiar – hugs, favourite food, much-loved stories, soothing music – interspersed with bouts of stimulation – outdoor play, finger painting, digging in the grass, chasing a ball. It is easier than handling the distress of older children but it is by no means easy on the parent. A 12-year-old explained to me recently, 'Adults expect us to behave like adults but treat us like children.' I understood that to mean that adults expect older children to soothe their own distress, regulate themselves, find ways to occupy themselves when it is convenient for the adult, but dismiss their views and opinions, refusing to take them seriously when it poses a challenge to the adult.

Children between the ages of six years and puberty are designed to learn and to move and certainly to learn by moving. When we shut this age group of children indoors, away from peer networks, outlets for creativity and energy, away from learning by fighting, falling, failing, we are shutting down a force of nature. Much like trying to shut down the wind, it will push back with force. When this development-design is interrupted, one of two things can happen. The urge to learn and move can either shut down or adapt (the quiet, listless, depressed child), or it can push back (the agitated, hyperactive, angry child). A 10-year-old may not be able to come up to you and say, 'I am aware that it is not possible to meet my friends but I really miss them and I miss playing in the park'; they may instead go quiet and lose their appetite. Or be stuck to a device: gaming. Or develop a habit of touching their genitals, wetting the bed or waking up with nightmares. Or they may be agitated, get aggressive and become difficult to calm. No one likes the aggressive child but the latter has more hope. Though it is not easy for the grown-ups who have to juggle work, virtual-school (which has huge problems of its own), home, attention-to-child, financial stress and COVID-anxiety at this time, this push-back is in fact a display of the child's resilience. It is demanding an outlet for its age-appropriate energy. From the perspective of the psychotherapist, the child who can be aggressive and protest has hope (Winnicott, 1986/1990). The quiet children are the ones we worry about the most.

This is usually the age group of under-14, for which we continue to get the maximum referrals in 2021. The first problem we face as a team with regard to this age group is that it is almost impossible to work effectively with them and have a trusting relationship built on a virtual platform. Nine-year-old Anamika is busy watching YouTube videos during our session, her eyes fixed on some other tab on the screen, while she insists she is talking to me. Thirteen-year-old Tarini is clearly playing Fortnite or Roblox while she multitasks and chatters away to the therapist at top speed, but about every-thing irrelevant and inane. This is not how therapy works. This inattention is not how any relationship works.

We all need a flesh-and-blood presence in order to connect to the reality of the other. On the screen, we are a two-dimensional presence, not a real person – no different from the YouTube videos or cartoons they watch. Our attention on them, our questions, our curiosity and our concern are all hypo-thetical. A 14-year-old summed it up when he said he preferred to have our sessions 'In Real Life' – as opposed to what, I wondered: imaginary? Fantasy? Because when the Zoom call is over, when the screen is closed, what happens to the person? What happens to the relationship when we have not breathed in the same room or experienced the other person's emotions as a bodily reality in front of us? Is there even a relationship between us?

Then there is our adolescent population, designed to disagree with adults and to bond with peers, but since the latter have now become virtual enti-ties, there is more of the first, less of the latter. Or we see symptoms of high anxiety. Adolescents are in the process of making relationships outside of their family and domestic arrangements. In addition, they are starting out on the toughest parts of human development – emotionally separating from parental figures and discovering their own selves. This process, technically called Identity Development (a phrase which unfortunately glosses over the emotional turmoil inherent in it), is difficult enough without the added bur-den of uncertainty of the future that older adolescents have to now face with the shadow of COVID. Leaving home and moving to another part of the country or to another continent was never easy, but now it comes with extra guilt and fear attached. Also 16- to 18-year-olds are struggling – unable to focus, suffering brain-fog, suicidal ideation, heart palpitations, insomnia; they are overwhelmed by the sheer weight of not-knowing and sometimes by rage. No wonder the tranquiliser or a gaming device or a joint, or even cutting themselves to let out blood, brings some calm.

When an adolescent knows what is at the base of their distress, our work is made easier. That rarely happens. Many of the 18- to 19-year-olds who have approached us do not link any of their distress to COVID. They disconnect it from external reality. Their distress is often minimized as their 'inability to be motivated' or 'everyone is handling it better than I am' or 'my friend has it harder so how can I admit to struggling'. There is also a hyperawareness of news, political upheaval and fight for rights in the external world (right to privacy, the farmers' protests, issues of citizenship and belonging, rights of the minority groups in India) with a jarring lack of compassion for the internal fight for rights. Then these young people do not know how to respond to our compassion towards them. It seems like an alien experience, which they both want and reject.

More often than not, adolescents come in apathetic and detached, therefore not really bothered or troubled by anything. They tend to be referred by a parent who can see the sabotage and self-harm. This apathy is rarely a problem to the teenager themselves since it is an effective solution to whatever distress they were originally feeling. Fifteen-year-old Ashish sat in front of me, slumped over, no muscle tone in his body, not making eye contact and responded with 'I don't know' to my question of what emotional difficulty he needed help with. After 20 minutes he could say that he often considered dying but he was not sure it was a problem he wanted help with. When I responded that it was certainly a problem for his family, who wanted him to be happy, he laughed a cynical, mirthless laugh and said, 'What does that even mean?' Eventually, we could reach the awareness that there was a part of him that did not want to die. It is not completely clear if that means he wants to live. We are still working on it.

Even 16- to 18-year-olds have come in, not making the link between their anxiety, low mood and the reality of having had their lives in lockdown. They minimize the impact of their losses by saying they are 'unmotivated' or 'just being lazy'. Between this minimization and judgement, our young people are expected to 'get on with it' and be productive, reach goals that have no meaning anymore to some (such as finishing grade 11). They are not even permitted to acknowledge that their life has come to a standstill.

***

In these years when our children have suffered multiple losses – of people, spaces, relationships and familiarity – it is not possible to move on to a conversation about gratitude without also acknowledging the losses, tempting as it may seem. Many of us are plagued by not being permitted to mourn because there is always someone else who has it worse, or 'we have so much to be grateful for' and 'we are really so blessed'. While this may also be true, 2020–2021 has also been the year of frozen dreams, especially for young people. Can we not make grief into a competitive sport? If we acknowledge individual, personal meaning, perhaps we can have permission to also mourn everything, everyone and every dream that died in 2020. Either/or thinking only shrinks us and makes for emotional poverty

Notes

1 This has been reproduced with permission from the child, now six years old, and his parents.
2 This section is taken from a previous publication by the first author (Paiva, 2020).
3 This section is taken from a previous publication by the first author (Paiva, 2022).

References

Bettelheim, B. (1987). The importance of play. *The Atlantic, 259*(3), 35–46.

Erikson, E. H. (1950). Toys and reasons. In *Childhood and Society*. W. W. Norton.

NCRB. (2019). *Suicides in India*. Retrieved November 8, 2021, from https://ncrb.gov.in/sites/default/files/Chapter-2-Suicides_2019.pdf

Paiva, N. D. (2018). *Love and rage: The inner worlds of children*. Yoda Press.

Paiva, N. D. (2020). Far away is the rainbow. *The Hindu.* www.thehindubusinessline.com/blink/cover/far-away-is-the-rainbow/article33090554.ece

Paiva, N. D. (2022). *Love and rage: The inner worlds of children* (2nd ed.). Yoda Press.

Rampal, N. (2020, September 4). More than 90,000 young adults died by suicide in 2019 in India: NCRB report. *India Today.* www.indiatoday.in/diu/story/ncrb-report-data-india-young-adults-suicide-2019-india-1717887-2020–09–02

Winnicott, D. W. (1990) Delinquency as a sign of hope. In *Home is where we start from; Essays by a psychoanalyst* (p. 90). W. W. Norton. (Original work published 1986)

2 Reflecting and integrating the inner child during challenging times

Rekha Sapra

Introduction

Even though literally speaking the inner child's existence may be a contentious issue, the concept of the inner child is metaphorically real. Like complexes in general, it is a psychological or phenomenological reality ('Complex (Psychology)', 2021), which is extraordinarily powerful. We were all children once and still have that child within us though as adults may not be aware of its presence. Many behavioural, emotional, and relationship difficulties have been found to have their roots due to this lack of conscious relatedness to our own inner child (Tulani, 2021). The longing of the 'inner child – for love, acceptance, protection, nurturance, understanding – remains the same today as when we were children' (Diamond, 2008). In spite of seeming to be successful adults, many situations can trigger a panic situation in us, leading to heavy breathing and a shaky demeanour. This may be the result of the unfulfilled needs of the inner child. Indeed, most mental disorders and destructive behaviour patterns are related to the unconscious part of the self. Judgement, decision making, motivation, and interpersonal attractions are the product of unconscious mental operations and take shape beyond our conscious awareness (Diamond, 2008).

Concept of the inner child in psychodynamic parlance

The inner child is a direct representation of oneself in early developmental years. The experiences in early childhood years play a decisive role during adulthood. Childhood is not always associated with fun, happiness, and carefree times for all. Childhood experiences for many abound with neglect, trauma, emotional pain, and vulnerability. In such cases the physical and psychological need for love, care, protection, and emotional support may remain unmet.

A child growing up in an accepting and loving environment with a safe space to voice his or her opinions, with no fear of ridicule or criticism, grows into a well-rounded personality, with high self-esteem, is resilient, and has good mental health. On the other hand, a child who is exposed to physical punishment frequently coupled with verbal and emotional abuse, is

DOI: 10.4324/9781003255895-3

not permitted to experience strong positive and negative emotions, or is not heard feels unsafe. Lack of physical affect in the form of hugs and cuddles and discouragement of spontaneous activities impacts the child negatively. As a consequence, this child feels insecure and unsafe.

Emotional neglect for prolonged periods may lead to low self-worth and self-esteem. The child learns to ignore her emotional needs and repress or hide those emotional needs which are associated with neglect. Emotional neglect may manifest itself in the form of mental, physical, or other health-related challenges. Emotional neglect leads to the inability to listen to or deal with one's emotions in a healthy manner.

Psychological neglect in the form of not 'listening' to the child in the early years, coupled with lack of nurture, hampers the social-emotional and psychological growth of the child. Abuse, ridicule, rejection, constant punishment, or ignoring the child leads to a lowered self-esteem and confidence in the child. As a consequence of this neglect, there can be anger issues, unresolved childhood trauma, inability to love, and so on. Addiction and neurosis may also overtly manifest themselves, giving a misguided sense of comfort and safety.

Every child has a right to feel safe, secure, and protected not only physically but also emotionally. Supporting a child on the emotional, psychological, and spiritual levels is critical for the mental, social, and emotional well-being of the child. When an individual does not feel safe for a long duration, a sense of endangerment lurks constantly. All parents may not have the ability to accept children unconditionally. Such experiences of neglect, trauma, and rejection leave a 'huge gaping wound in the psyche' (Davis, 2020) and the child may feel repressed unknowingly. The inner child is the part of our psyche that retains its liveliness, innocence, and genuine surprise and these are crucial components of childhood behaviour. A healthy inner child remains connected, excited with curiosity and inquisitiveness, so characteristic of the early years.

The most common characteristics of an unsafe environment are when the child is made to feel that it's not okay for her to put forward her opinion or is punished for voicing her opinion. The child is not encouraged to play or indulge in playful spontaneous activities. If the child does not have a sense of belonging to the family or is not permitted to be herself, coupled with lack of physical contact with the child in the form of hugging, cuddling, or kissing, an unsafe and threatening space is created in the child's psyche.

A supportive and a non-shaming, non-judgemental space is needed in therapeutic sessions, which the inner child has not received due to neglect, abuse, rejection, or abandonment during early years, to integrate the wounded inner child. The important issues which need to be addressed in any therapy session should focus on the timeline during early years when the child experienced repetitive negative emotions in the environment: how the individual felt as a child and to connect to the feelings and emotions then experienced. The constant feeling of anxiety, worrying extensively, trust issues, harsh criticism of the self, doubting the self, and lacking the concept of a personal space are some of the indicators of an inner child who craves for love and nurturance.

The symptoms of emotional neglect during childhood show up in adulthood as numbing out or lack of connect with one's feelings; a feeling of hollowness or something missing inside, low self-esteem; and trying to be a perfectionist, high sensitivity to rejection (Webb, 2012). Emotional neglect by the caregivers may not always be because of any bad intention. Maybe the parents themselves had a rejected or neglected childhood. The consequences of child abuse and neglect may vary depending on the susceptibility of the individual to adverse outcomes and factors like family, parenting, the social context of the child, severity of the neglect, chronicity, and the timing of the neglect. All these factors impact an individual to varying degrees. The neural, behavioural, and biological outcomes may vary for different individuals. Severe early deprivation has been found to lead to deficits in attention regulation (Petersen et al., 2014). The inner scarred child never goes away. Even during adulthood, the inner child makes its presence felt where a feeling of persistent unhappiness prevails and the perception of the world as a dangerous and horrible place keeps lurking at the back of the mind. A massive gaping wound opens in the psyche, which is extremely painful, and as a consequence, it is repressed (Kneisl, 1991). Emotional neglect during childhood may also result in lack of personal boundaries. The individual feels that she is being manipulated, controlled, exploited, or dominated. Confused boundaries result in co-dependency, toxicity, and one-sided relationships. Strong and clear personal boundaries are critical for healthy relationships, self-esteem, and a positive self-image. Sometimes parents can be bad role models, with co-dependency in family dynamics; they may reinforce and equate love with 'acceptable behaviour'. This results in lack of personal boundaries as adults.

Healthy personal boundaries make a person empowered and attract healthy and supportive friends and partners. The individual has the feeling of being valued and heard by others and emotional and personal well-being is experienced. An inner child with many insecurities, when grown into an adult, is like a child left alone in a new environment without parental support or intervention. The child feels lost and confused. An adult with an unhealed or wounded inner child displays emotionally immature behaviour has issues related to career and relationships, and her decision-making skills are adversely impacted. This condition gets worse under challenging situations. The challenges may be internal or external threats.

The pandemic and its impact on the inner child

The COVID-19 pandemic has proved to be a prolonged and severe crisis facing humanity in recent years. The extended quarantine periods have come with a plethora of psychological burdens and neuro-psychiatric consequences which can have a long-term negative impact. The cramped and limited space available to most people, coupled with other stresses, insecurities, and fears, has resulted in higher levels of physical and verbal aggression as well increase in cases of punishment and domestic violence (Ghosh et al., 2020).

The psychological burden of the pandemic, coupled with its psychosocial ill effects, needs to be considered in the light of the inner child/children and its long-term consequences for future adolescents and adults. The response of adults with a wounded inner child to the pandemic needs to be revisited by psychologists and other mental health professionals and many more research investigations need to be undertaken in order to assess the long-term consequences of home quarantine for an extended duration. The absence of social interaction with the outside world needs to be explored at length. The positive role of the social media in enabling people to interact on various virtual platforms has been like a ray of hope for many, though this cannot be a substitute for actual one-to-one interaction.

Psychological aggression and physical punishments can leave permanent wounds in the form of an impaired brain and poor development of the psyche. These may result in higher psychosomatic and neuro-psychiatric disorders as well as higher instances of substance abuse and suicidal tendencies (United Nations, 2020).

The closure of schools has resulted in space outside the home becoming inaccessible to children along with the consequent educational and learning limitations. Limited or lack of access to free space for children, both physically and psychologically, does have a negative impact on the developing child. This window of freedom offered by schools being shut down and the scope of interactions giving psychological solace and emotional outlet being impacted leads to the feeling of captivity being all-pervasive.

Increased incidences of child abuse, teenage promiscuity due to increased stress levels and close proximity, high school dropout rates because of the financial restraints of the family and loss of earning opportunities, high-risk behaviour, and increase in child labour are some of the concerns with associated potential risks (ILO, 2020). Both children and adults who are facing anxieties, sexual exploitation, and economic burden have a higher risk of being impacted in any adverse situation, and the pandemic can be compared to a crisis situation for human existence (United Nations, 2020).

The lack of conscious relatedness to our own inner child results in behavioural, emotional, and relationship deficits and other mental health issues. The wounded child needs 'reassurance' and 'acceptance' so that he or she can come out of hiding. The wounded inner child must be able to trust that, as an adult, we are able to empathize and are there for him or her for support (Davis, 2020; 'How to Nurture and Reparent Your Inner Child,' 2019).

More rigorous longitudinal research studies need to be undertaken in order to understand the impact of the pandemic on adults with an existing wounded inner child as well as the formation of the inner child/children during stressful situations in childhood vis-à-vis parenting, parental relationships, and other contributing factors in terms of adjustment of children to their personal and social spaces.

Healing the inner child

The biggest challenge one faces as a therapist is to identify the inner child and start working on it. The healing process can be initiated only when the existence of the inner child is acknowledged and recognized. The first and foremost important aspect in healing is accepting things or persons which caused the pain in childhood and bringing the hurt out to help it find an outlet in the form of verbalization or an emotional outburst. Also, it is important to listen to feelings which must have been aroused during situations that trigger strong emotions or discomfort. The process may involve opening old wounds and anger experienced when the needs were unmet, leading to a sense of abandonment, rejection, or feelings of guilt, shame, and anxiety that must have been dominant during those unpleasant and threatening experiences.

Mindful self-awareness brings about its own physical and mental health benefits for the individual. Self-awareness in a mindful way can be achieved by paying focused attention to one's feelings. This facilitates the identification of the trigger and makes the person more comfortable with unwanted emotions. One needs to experience both positive and negative emotions. These are meant to be experienced and expressed. Repressed emotions express themselves in many harmful ways. Accepting negative emotions as well as leaving the door open so as to experience emotions and feelings in a healthy and accepting way is part of one's mental and experiential repertoire.

Healing the inner child involves clearing the emotional baggage of childhood by way of grieving and acknowledging the wounds that have been suffered. To change behaviour patterns, it is essential to clear the emotions – to release unexpressed grief with its pent-up rage, shame, terror, and pain from those feeling places which exist within the individual (Raypole, 2021).

There is a strong need to nurture, love, and rescue the inner child. This can be achieved by accepting and honouring the child who suffered in childhood. This is crucial so that the person is able to love and accept herself. The owning and honouring of the child's experiences and feelings helps to release the emotional grief energy that we as adults still carry around.

Emotions are an integral part of a human being. Both positive and negative emotions need to be acknowledged, identified, and expressed appropriately. Needs must be identified and are critical to developing an emotional vocabulary. Emotion regulation, a very essential life skill, needs to be reinforced from early childhood years (Sapra, 2015). It is very important to be compassionate with oneself and not be overcritical.

Conclusion

What exactly is our inner child? The inner child is the child we once were, which did not grow up. The inner child holds memories, emotions, as well as good and bad experiences. The negative and harmful words and actions of caregivers make the child feel threatened and unsafe. The wounded inner child influences and moulds the adult personality, exercising immense power over the relationships and decisions of the adult.

The inner child who resides within our subconscious mind wants to enjoy, have fun, and play. This inner child can help and act as a buffer in stressful situations. This inner child is a person within who needs healing, support, and reinforcement through skills and coping tools. Connect with the inner child can be established to heal the wounded inner child's happiness and the feeling of being loved. The inner child needs a healthy outlet in the form of creative, spontaneous, and fun activities.

References

Complex (Psychology). (2021, August 12). *Wikipedia.* https://en.wikipedia.org/w/index.php?title=Complex_(psychology)&oldid=1037102305

Davis, S. (2020, July 13). The wounded inner child. *CPTSD Foundation.* https://cptsdfoundation.org/2020/07/13/the-wounded-inner-child/

Diamond, S. A. (2008, June 7). Essential secrets of psychotherapy: The inner child. *Psychology Today.* www.psychologytoday.com/us/blog/evil-deeds/200806/essential-secrets-psychotherapy-the-inner-child

Ghosh, R., Dubey, M. J., Chatterjee, S., & Dubey, S. (2020). Impact of COVID-19 on children: special focus on the psychosocial aspect. *Minerva Pediatrics*, 72(3), 226–235. https://doi.org/10.23736/S0026-4946.20.05887-9

How to nurture and reparent your inner child. (2019, October 25). Retrieved August 20, 2021, from www.gstherapycenter.com/blog/2019/10/25/how-to-nurture-and-reparent-your-inner-child

ILO. (2020). *Covid-19 impact on child labour and forced labour: The response of the IPEC+ flagship programme.* www.ilo.org/wcmsp5/groups/public/-ed_norm/-ipec/documents/publication/wcms_745287.pdf

Kneisl, C. R. (1991). Healing the wounded, neglected inner child of the past. *Nursing Clinics of North America*, 26(3), 745–755. https://pubmed.ncbi.nlm.nih.gov/1891407/

Petersen, A. C., Joseph, J., & Feit, M. (Eds.). (2014). *New directions in child abuse and neglect research; Committee on Child Maltreatment Research, Policy and Practice for next decade: Phase II, Board on Children Youth and Families.* National Academic Press. www.ncbi.nlm.nih.gov/books/NBK195985

Raypole, C. (2021, October 21). 8 Ways to start healing your inner child. *Healthline.* www.healthline.com/health/mental-health/inner-child-healing

Sapra, R. (2015, October). *Intervention strategies to enhance social-emotional learning in young children.* Unpublished manuscript. Major Research Project supported by UGC.

Tulani, S. (2021, July 3). *Reparenting the inner child.* Pahoti Wellness. https://pahotiwellness.com/blog/reparenting-the-inner-child/

United Nations. (2020, April 15). *Policy brief: The impact of Covid-19 on children.* https://unsdg.un.org/sites/default/files/2020-04/160420_Covid_Children_Policy_Brief.pdf

Webb, J. (2012). *Running on empty: Overcome your childhood neglect.* Morgan James Publishing.

3 Psychic withdrawal to dreaming

Gliding the spectrum during COVID-19

Neetu Sarin

A truth that the ongoing pandemic has established is that no two days are the same. One morning, I may wake up despondent, and the next, I am hyper-creative and making a three-course meal and putting up photos on social media. Some mornings, I wake up rested and relieved at not having to go out anywhere, while on others I look longingly at my old photos, yearning for the time I will be able to meet friends and step out.

Just as there are multiple versions of our days and nights, we have within ourselves, a multiplicity of emotional self-states (Sturgeon, 1953; Bromberg, 2001 etc.) To a non-psychological observer, these may appear as moods or emotions. However, they are really varying self-states or mini-personhoods within us, an amalgamation of which makes us 'ME'. Under ordinary conditions, we distribute the airtime to these varying self-states fairly, dividing them up into professional self, personal self, social self and private or secret self. Since the onset of the coronavirus pandemic, the sanity-inducing boundary between these selves is blurred, and all these parts are expected to work from the same geographical location – our screens, a feat that requires a lot of psychological sophistication and spiritual elevation.

In this chapter, I will make an attempt to urge us to use the thread of 'dreaming' as the unitary thread that weaves the fragmented parts of ourselves. However, before I go there, I would like to share a few observations on the pandemic self. In the last 15 months, one way in which we have tried to maintain continuity between our pre-pandemic and post-pandemic selves is by adopting virtual reality like never before. As a desperate way of maintaining contact with each other, we have been using the myriad online platforms in vogue. We tell ourselves that, perhaps, we can compensate for our physical caging by going anywhere virtually. So, isn't it great, then? Yet, why is it so difficult to be in this lockdown?

In a very short time, we have traversed several self-states: that of terror, helplessness, rage, omnipotence and denial. Perhaps, the 'turning inwards' necessitated by the pandemic is a powerful antidote to the manic productivity of society (see Altman, 2020). At the outset, I want to distinguish between this 'turning inwards' and a more severe form of detachment called psychic withdrawal. Psychoanalysts like Steiner (1993), Klein (1959), Winnicott

DOI: 10.4324/9781003255895-4

(1971) and Bion (1965) have spoken extensively of at least one part of our personality that is inaccessible to others, which we keep privately for our own thoughts, musings and dreams. Not only is this part private but it is also sealed off from inquiry or curiosity from others. A very ordinary example is a daydream; while suddenly listening to a podcast or some music, you may find yourself zoning out and fantasizing about the evening's dinner, or a memory of your sixteenth birthday. These repetitive, irrelevant parts of our life are hardly ever shared with anyone else, not only because they are precious but mostly because we do not think there is much relevance to them. This everyday withdrawal, when in the shadows of a trauma, can be propelled into pathological proportions which, while being experienced, may be transformed into dreaming.

A 65-year-old gentleman, who came to see me for therapy, told me that he was single and happily unmarried. Elaborating, he presented a long and detailed account of the 'agony marriage is, how two people have to live with each other, how one never has the bathroom to oneself, lack of space' and so on. I thought to myself, that was a lot of imagination for an experience he had never had! Sometimes, we fantasize so that we never have to live the experience, wherein fantasy takes over reality, and what we imagine becomes the driver of our decision making.

For most of us, there is an ongoing negotiation between reality and imagination. We are always looking for facts and clarity of instructions from our parents, our teachers, the government and others. At the same time, human beings have a remarkable inner agency that allows them to negotiate the uncertainty of external reality via an *inner unconscious fantasy*, our ability to mould reality according to our wishes, desires, historical locations, gender, class and so on. In our internal unconscious fantasy, we keep spinning a web of stories, creating for ourselves an equilibrium between anxiety and rest. This negotiation may reflect itself in making plans for when the pandemic ends or asking our friends, 'Do you think we will still be making our own meals once all this ends?' These are all creative imaginations, or reveries (Bion, 1965), and must be thought of as mental states in which conscious and unconscious communications are transferred between two people, without any tangible concreteness. These transient, seemingly silly thoughts are powerful vehicles of unconscious communication. Bion (1965) called them the alpha function, the part which lends meaning, that is simultaneously processing the present as well as imagining a future. *So even though it may seem that we are helpless in the face of the pandemic, our inner worlds are not so helpless*, a point I will return to when I talk of dreaming later in the chapter.

The spaces *between* the real and virtual

To begin with, I want to create a psychological landscape for those of us who have seamlessly glided into the virtual world. Before the virus struck, we would use the Internet as an *alternative* to real-time dialogue and connections. However, now, virtual gatherings are the *only* or predominant mode of operating! Is it possible that instead of connecting us to each other, virtual reality may be taking us further away from each other? Let me explain.

Real versus virtual. Original versus copy. No longer is virtual reality an augmentation of the real world, but an alternative to it.

When we are in person with another human being, we gather a sense of three-dimensionality, a depth of human experience (Meltzer, 1975). Body style, posture, gait, mobility and 'static-ness' are carefully noticed. What is at one end of the body ego formation is the experience of mimesis: a form of identification that involves gestures, style of being and styles of speech. It takes forward Lacan's (1953) idea of mirroring, bringing to the picture the corporeal body that mimics. Mimesis, the experience of merging the self in the experience of the other, is an experience both active and passive, creating body ego through the use of the other, but an other who is an active seer, not neutral. The embodiment of experience is the foundation for discovering the otherness of the other. When a three-dimensional experience exists, there is a 'you', 'me' and 'something else'. This *something else* is very crucial, even if unnameable, and the intimacy between two people depends on how much they are willing to find out what this 'something else' is. Corporeal bodies allow the creation of a three-dimensional world, allowing us to think of emotional problems as not merely existing on either one or the other side of a 'paper-thin object' (Meltzer, 1975). The world seems full of potential spaces and emotional containers (Bion, 1965).

The virtual world, on the other hand, provides us with one or two-dimensionality, not three, which gives us an *illusion* of intimacy, but the third, the 'something else', is missing. Meltzer (1975) writes:

> A linear relationship of time-distance between self and object would give rise to a world which had a fixed centre in the self, and a system of radiating lines having direction and distance to objects which were conceived as potentially attractive or repellent.
>
> (p. 224)

In a one- or two-dimensional world, gratification and differentiation with persons/objects seems undifferentiated and geared towards soothing and self-placating – something like an autistic state of mind. The self then becomes impoverished in imagination, even though intelligent in perception. The more we rely on screens to keep us alive, the more depleted we become in imagination. We are then left with little-to-no means for constructing (in thought) objects, events and situations different from those actually experienced. The leaner the dimensionality, the thinner the realm of an internal mind where fantasy can operate. Hence, the question is whether virtual closeness brings us closer or merely gives us an illusion of closeness. This is probably why, besides the strain of staring into a screen, we come away feeling exhausted.

The disappearing body and dread

Neuroscientists have been studying the impact of simulating bodies for over a decade (Haans et al., 2008; Shaefer et al., 2009; Slater et al., 2010). After a sufficient amount of simulation, the brain can be tricked into taking ownership of a body or body part that is not ours. These experiments found that by making people wear headsets, empathy for not-mine bodies could be generated (Haans et al., 2008; Metral, 2017). This indicates that, even though it is virtual, the necessary boundary between two bodies can collapse. When in real-time contact, we are aware of the contours of our body, its boundary and its limits. However, with continuous virtual exposure, the brain can believe that what we see on the screen is ours, which might explain why so many of us find online interactions addictive and tiring – *our tiredness is a constant attempt on our part to orient ourselves: 'are you looking at me, or someone else; should I speak now or should I wait for my turn?'*

In the virtual world, we are far more porous to influence and suggestion than in the physical world. Is this possibly because we do not have avenues for body cues to either warn us or encourage us?

I do not mean to demonize the virtual space but only to proceed with caution towards the way the Internet can disembody an individual's history and transience. I can be anyone or anything without a body barrier. When we are with other humans corporeally, we are vibrantly negotiating what is reality and what lies in our imagination. A screen bypasses this psychic work and presents to us only a projection of our internal worlds. When I have a virtual meeting, I am bound to imagine the space my colleague is sitting in: what does her house look like, does she have pets or is she rich? All that should remain in the private domain becomes oddly public, which in future may give me an illusion that there is no privacy in human matters.

Furthermore, the negotiation between reality and phantasy makes us develop psychologically, as it involves emotional labour, an emotional exercise. It provides the foundation for a contact barrier (Breuer & Freud, 1895/1955) between the world and ourselves. The virtual world robs us of this labour and growth. 'As long as we think of this virtual reality as temporary it is fine', we tell ourselves. But our psyches do not work so rationally. Once we get hooked to this easy way of negotiating life, we are likely to find going back tough.

Perhaps we are all living on the control-helplessness spectrum, known in psychoanalysis as 'dread' (Mitchell, 1993; Eigen, 1999 etc.). The sense of cataclysmic events happening to the self as it was beginning to stabilize never fully leaves. Breakdowns are inevitable, although the quality of support in its wake redeems us. 'The atmospheric tone surrounding breakdown can drive one further down, or lift one through' (Eigen, 1999). We are all turning to our screens in the hope of this redemption, to protect ourselves from complete isolation. If we do not use this forum, we may die of isolation, and if we do, lack of emotional vibrancy would be a death sentence.

I highly suspect that once all this is over, we may actually need to hold a collective debriefing – how to behave with each other as if we are not living on screens. Even though the subliminal lesson during the pandemic is to slow down, introspect, we are undoing a reality that has the potential of teaching us what infants need to learn as part of growing up: *I am not the king of the world* – omnipotence. The pandemic is a huge democrat; it has affected all humans similarly with dread and anxiety. In the matrix of life and death in which fate rules, all men and women are mere playthings.

The pandemic is also democratic in rendering hope: 'slow down, step out less, and talk less.' If we are to think of our lockdown locations as a metaphor of our beings, then we are being invited to discover those parts of our being that have largely remained neglected or untouched. Just like I suddenly see my neighbours using their terraces and balconies, we are unexpectedly in touch with our rich internal worlds. And this is the point where I come to the dreaming potential activated by the pandemic.

The dreaming potential: Portal to healing

In dreams, we experience a somatic flexibility, a characteristic common to virtual reality and dreams! We can be whoever we wish (and sometimes dread) to be, without having to put in any conscious effort. The thrill of speed and chameleon-like alteration of selfhood makes our dreams the richest motif of our internal worlds.

I use *dreams and the process of dreaming* in the hope that looking at our situation through the lens of dreams may provide a useful orientation into the strangeness of our shared catastrophe. Many of my patients report an increase in their night dreams. Those who are not in therapy also seem to be reporting dreams. The psychoanalytic tool of dream analysis is no longer confined to the consulting room, as every household may have at least one conversation such as 'I had a bizarre dream last night'.

For us psychoanalysts, this is very good news! Just as we are now introspecting upon the impact of human destruction of ecosystems, we also need to mourn that we have destroyed the habitat for our dreams. Modern life is a habitat for doing, with little structural sanctity for *being*, compromising both dreams and night. Day and night no longer have much sanctity, which is why this recent appearance of dreams demands special attention.

For as long as we can remember we have been mystified by the meaning of images that pass through us while sleeping. Are dreams still the royal road to the unconscious? How do they play a role in our daily interactions and our clinical work? Do we need a different conception of dreams and thereby the unconscious? I often wonder where my mind is when I sleep. And how are my dreams so lucid, colourful and rested when my waking life is full of unrest and anxiety? Some dreams are mundane but some are hallucinatory masterpieces.

Dreams have been given a sanctity in ancient cultures. Kings and queens have often relied on their dreams to make decisions; family members often think of dreams as ancestors passing on their wisdom or as divine inspiration (Hughes, 2000). Sometimes dreams appear scary and like curses, as in a nightmare or a divine presence, creating worries that we did not even know we had.

How is it that in the face of this enormous giant called COVID, our dream life has in fact gone up? Perhaps, when the noise of external reality goes up, psychic reality also steps up to keep pace. The compass of unconscious thinking is kept alive in dreaming. While this plague comes at a huge human cost, this invisible virus is also redeeming human beings for, ironically, we are being forced to accept the punyness of the human race in the face of death, and we must undo the damage caused by our omnipotent greed. And this is where dreams might save us.

However, one also wonders if we shouldn't be traumatized instead of dreaming. Here are a few possible explanations for this:

1   There is an intimate connection between helplessness and magic. We all believed in magic when we were children. And then we became agentic and stopped believing in magic. The more COVID drives us towards helplessness, the more our faith in magic may grow! The primitive part of our mind that believes in magic, which is driven by the logic of the heart and not the rational mind, the part which operates from a preverbal state may be at work more in these times. As the virus persists, we have more and more opportunities to be illogical, less oppressed by the demands of society. Our collective psyche may relax and the imaginative psyche, locked down upon due to modern living and social censors, may finally be coming out to play, like the wild animals we are seeing on empty roads of our cities.

2   A receding of external distraction may allow us to spend more time thinking of ourselves, spend time in our own company. The company does not have to be pleasant, but it gives data to our mind to generate thoughts. The potential benefit of catastrophic change occurs first at an individual level and, by so doing, paves the way towards the process of mourning past losses. Some of my patients report that a greater loneliness has forced them to make friends with their own selves. Some report picking up from their bookshelves novels they had never noticed. A dizziness of stimulation doesn't allow dreaming.

3   Given the democratic way in which all countries of the world are feeling helpless, our minds are finally relying on the authority of our inner minds and not only on external leaders.

4   For many individuals, with the reminder that there is nowhere to go, we may be actually remembering more dreams than before. A transitional period between self-states becomes possible when manic activity (pertaining to modern-day living, not necessarily individual mania) is reduced, allowing ourselves to be created at the same time that we try to articulate that creation. Could we then use this time for not

self-improvement and expertise but to turn inwards and use the beauty of our unconscious minds to create aliveness and vibrancy in these uncertain times?

The paradigm of dreams *reflecting* our unconscious began with Freud (1900/1953), whose most cooperative patient was himself. Working with hysteric patients, Freud discovered the 'repressed unconscious': the part of the psyche that forgets, usually one's own sexual and sometimes one's demonic parts. As we read *Studies on Hysteria* (1895), we see the work of the unconscious. The unconscious is not simply a storehouse where the abandoned, dirty, unacceptable parts of our psyche reside but a rich process by which our psyche negotiates with the real world outside of us like our families, teachers, friends and lovers. It's also the *meaning-making instrument*, which allows us an understanding of what is happening to us from inside (not only as a response to stimuli but a plethora of images, desires, fact-finding and creative pursuits that we encounter within ourselves). In short, we have come a long way from the *understanding of the unconscious as a storehouse of the repressed. It's also the site of infinite creativity*. The question is no longer whether the dream has this or that meaning but what we can know about the human race going through this calamity through dreams.

In these deeply fragmented times, I suggest that we focus on *working with dreams, and not on them*. Why do I call these times fragmented?, you may ask. As we are left without the ability to use necessary defences in relationships, little capacity to link the sequence of everyday events meaningfully, and sometimes a diminished capacity to distinguish inner fantasy from reality, fragmentation, indigestible and untranslatable life, is what envelopes us.

My effort is to suggest that dreams are not only nocturnal healing but a significant parameter of unconscious waking life. As someone who is interested in Japanese authors like Murakami, or Portuguese poets like Fernando Pessoa, who allude to the thinly veiled 'other worlds', I can't help but look at the dreaming in daily life, in relationships and in waking states. Dreams help us symbolize, but symbolization also depends on the capacity to dream.

Let us start with Freud not only because he discovered psychoanalysis but because he allowed himself to be discovered, thereby setting up a discipline with *self-inquiry as the cornerstone of knowledge*. When Freud theorized *The Interpretation of Dreams* (1900/1953), he made a major shift from the physical to the mental. He starts with a hydraulic energy model (energy build-up during the day finds the necessary discharge during the night in dreams) but ends up with an interpretive, hermeneutic model (dreams tell us how we are making sense of our lives). For me, this is the most significant part of the dream work: the *shift* in the psyche when something begins to make sense. Not better, not worse, simply different.

In analysis, we invite the patient to enter the maze of these dreams and find their way out. Dreams are sites of research; images in dreams act as symbols, the deconstruction of which is the work of the therapeutic pair. As one of my patients asked me, 'Do you think I am crying in the dream because I cannot cry in reality?' It is possible, very possible, but I think we would be reducing the aesthetic quality of dreams if we only look at their wish fulfilment or discharging nature. As the Italian psychoanalyst Civitarese (2014) says, 'Dreams are outside the economy of usefulness.' If we are to dream, we will have to suspend the need to understand them logically, and reason is the first casualty of COVID-19. The grief, the loss, not only feels unsurmountable but illogical and inexplicable. How do we explain people who are fit, young and seemingly resourceful falling prey to this deadly virus? Why would large congregations of people amass together knowing how fatal it could be? No, logic does not describe the pandemic.

I borrow here from the French analyst Laplanche (1999), who stressed the unmistakable potency of the process of *aprés-coup*, indicating the nonlinear nature of time. The pandemic, and the accompanying political, economic and climate crisis, is, perhaps, opening the portal to repressed and unmourned traumatic events of the past. Losses of loved ones due to the virus bring up deep feelings of loss from the past. The ghastly event of COVID-19 has pixelated human experiences: hazy, unfocused, unclear, yet there. There is some amount of helplessness that comes with being human. It has opened up old wounds, which exacerbate the impact of the pandemic, making it not simply a tragedy but trauma. The 'dreaming' then would be to embrace the inevitable forms of helplessness in all of us. The more all of us, especially the analyst, accept the helplessness that comes with being human, the easier it would be to use the process of dreaming.

However, if I use Bion's idea (Aguayo & Malin, 1967) that dream life can be viewed as a place to which we can go in our sleep, then we can turn our attention fully to this internal world for the process of dreaming produces creative meaning that can then be employed in life and relationships in the external world.

Perhaps it would not be too presumptuous to say that a certain inner withdrawal is not only helpful but necessary today. Reflecting on our inner selves, through meditation, therapy, and music, gives as an opportunity to sequester ourselves from modern-day multiple selves and return home to the voice of our inner selves. Before poise comes madness, and if we tolerate the madness around and in us just a little while, peace is around the corner. We are on the edge of a collective transformation, where the *aprés-coup* can seem horrifying and terrorizing but also carries the potential to heal old wounds.

References

Aguayo, J. R., & Malin, B. D. (1967). *Wilfred Bion: Los Angeles seminars and supervisions*. Karnac.

Altman, N. (2020). *White privilege: Psychoanalytic perspectives*. Routledge.

Bion, W. R. (1965). *Transformations: Change from learning to growth*. Basic Books.

Breuer, J., & Freud, S. (1955). Studies on hysteria. In J. Strachey (Ed. and Trans.), *The standard edition of the complete psychological works of Sigmund Freud* (Vol. II). Hogarth Press. (Original work published 1895).

Bromberg, P. M. (2001). *Standing in the spaces: Essays on clinical process, trauma, and dissociation*. Analytic Press.

Civitarese, G. (2014). *The necessary dream: New theories and techniques of interpretation in psychoanalysis* (I. Harvey, Trans., 1st ed.). Routledge.

Eigen, M. (1999). *Toxic nourishment*. Karnac.

Freud, S. (1953). Interpretation of dreams. In J. Strachey (Ed. and Trans.), *The standard edition of the complete psychological works of Sigmund Freud* (Vol. IV). Hogarth Press. (Original work published 1900).

Haans, A., Ijsselsteijn, W. A., & de Kort, Y. A. W. (2008). The effect of similarities in skin texture and hand shape on perceived ownership of a fake limb. *Body Image, 5*(4), 389–394.

Hughes, J. D. (2000). Dream interpretation in ancient civilizations. *Dreaming, 10*(1), 7–18. https://doi.org/10.1023/A:1009447606158

Klein, M. (1959). Our adult world and its roots in infancy. In *Envy and gratitude and other works* (pp. 1946–1963). Free Press.

Lacan, J. (1953). Back to Freud. In *Seminar I: The seminar of Jacques Lacan*. W. W. Norton.

Laplanche, J. (1999). *Essays on otherness*. Routledge.

Meltzer, D. (1975). *Explorations in autism*. Payot.

Metral, M., Gonthier, C., Luyat, M., & Guerraz, M. (2017). Body schema illusions: A study of the link between the rubber hand and kinaesthetic mirror illusions through individual differences. *Biomed Research International, 2017*, Article 6937328. https://doi.org/10.1155/2017/6937328

Mitchell, S. A. (1993). *Hope and dread in psychoanalysis*. Basic Books.

Shaefer, M., Heinz,. J., & Rotte, M. (2009). My third arm: Shifts in topography of the somatosensory homunculus predict feeling of an artificial supernumerary arm. *Human Brain Mapping, 30*(5). https://doi.org/10.1002/hbm.20609

Slater, M., Spanlang, B., Sanchez-Vives, M., & Blanke, O. (2010). First person experience of body transfer in virtual reality. *PLoS One,* (5).

Steiner, J. (1993). *Psychic retreats: Pathological organizations in psychotic, neurotic and borderline patients*. Routledge. https://doi.org/10.4324/9780203359839

Sturgeon, T. (1953). *More than human*. Farrar, Straus & Young.

Winnicott, D. W. (1971). Dreaming, fantasizing and living. In *Playing and reality*. Routledge.

4 Against psychoanalytic form

Witnessing the unconscious with Lacan

Ahmad Fuad Rahmat

Objective

This chapter considers psychoanalysis's relevance for a COVID world by revisiting Lacan's account of analysts as witnesses to the unconscious. The significance of witnessing is premised on the unconscious's indeterminate quality, namely, how it is only met at the failure of knowledge. Consequently, to be a witness to the unconscious is to usher the analysand's singularity where knowledge lacks rather than to generate more meaning to consume. Applied to the present, analysts could well serve as witnesses to lost speech. Where the rush for cures and clarity throws us further into the daily tug-of-war between relevant and expired knowledge, analysis can be where singular voices silenced by the engulfing COVID emergency could be heard.

It is less noted, however, that Lacan encountered this limit by situating the present, the high point of modern science, as a moment in the longer unfolding of a historical crisis. This began in the chasm of knowledge left in the wake of Europe's scientific revolution, where the fall of medieval metaphysics was met with the proliferation of knowledge that intensified, rather than pacified, anxieties of the unknown. The destructive and crisis-ridden nature of the modern world is essentially rooted to the denial of this chasm, for which various infrastructures imposing universal and homogenising solutions – from science and capitalism as well as religious and racial fanaticism – emerge. Indeed, the aim of analysis is in many ways to remove the analysand from this need to master knowledge. So, in saying that we are witnesses to the unconscious, Lacan is not just describing what an analyst does. To witness lack is to also embody psychoanalysis's socio-historical role as a radical intervention against modernity's totalising and imperial drive.

COVID, however, allows us to explore a crucial implication to this claim. For Lacan, the institutionalisation of psychoanalysis is symptomatic of the problem psychoanalysis was supposed to address. It stems from the establishment assumption that the analyst could and should handle the transference objectively, an assumption that erroneously positions the analyst as an authority of knowledge. This possibility of being above discord is at

DOI: 10.4324/9781003255895-5

the core of anxieties to ensure that psychoanalysis is a legitimate science. Lacan sees it as contrary to the radicality of the Freudian project which was found where science arrived at its epistemic limits as it could not come to grips with the unconscious. It is with an affinity to the Real location of this discovery – at the margins of knowledge – that Lacan believes psychoanalysis has no other definition than lack. But taking the radicality of this event seriously requires that the analyst too is situated in those margins. Analytic witnessing then is not to be done dispassionately but from the mire of the transference where knowledge, especially the analyst's knowledge, fails upon a contingent encounter with lack. Psychoanalysis requires no form other than a loyalty to this moment.

This chapter is of course not the venue to debate Lacan's stance on analytic institutionalisation. It suffices, however, to draw out a present-day provocation out of his project, namely, how psychoanalysts should position themselves in the COVID era when the bellicose nature of knowledge – its geopolitical and epistemic contests – will be more obvious than ever. With Lacan we are able to see this not as a sudden aberration caused by the overwhelming wave of COVID panic but the global exposure of the long-standing historical coupling of knowledge and anxiety, or the failure to reduce knowledge to a handmaiden for our deepest fears. If this is the case, then psychoanalysts should similarly wonder if their clinic is just staging another moment in the contest or if they are witnessing something other to it – a witnessing Lacan asserts they can only do in lack. This requires us to remain in the threshold of knowledge's failure. Witnessing the unconscious is the extent to which the analyst is willing to desire difference in the moment he realised the adequacy of his knowledge. It is a question of resolve rather than ideals. Consequently, to see analysis as a historical practice is to pursue newer possibilities of witnessing, as the scramble for knowledge will certainly intensify.

If there is another reason to think about witnessing, it is also because it is insufficiently appreciated in Lacanian discourse. On the rare occasions when witnessing is discussed, it is under the ambit of the analyst's desire or presence. While the analyst's desire and presence are different instantiations of the same process, the more understated notion of witnessing stresses the unique nature of the 'conclusion' to the liquidation, namely, when the analyst comes to realise his lack through a certain unexpected defect in his understanding of the analytic situation. There is an evental chance element that the verb conveys more effectively in any case, as we generally identify as 'witnesses' only to more exceptional occurrences. This could be upheld somewhat as a crucial analytic feature to be considered when the COVID era has compelled many questions about psychoanalytic ideals.

With that in mind, my overview of Lacan will entail two things. The first is the historical dimension of the psychoanalytic subject, since Lacan sees modernity as entailing the antagonisms of knowledge-accumulation in the failure to overcome lack. The second is to show how this failure is confronted in the transference, namely, the ensuing liquidation of the subject-supposed-to-know, as the analysand embodies lack where the analyst's aura of authority also dissolves. Key in the comparison across the two sections is where the ordered hyper-rational world is met with a torsion into the unexpected in the clinic. The way Lacan turns to the Cartesian cogito to describe this process will be key as it elucidates the basis on which Lacan theorises the 'moment' the analyst is to witness.

The point of witnessing is not the effectiveness of technique or the application of a theory but the eventuality of lack. In many ways this eventuality of lack is witnessed where knowledge doesn't apply, where the analyst and analysand realise their investment in its hollowness – its fundamentally imaginary, rather than substantive, quality. With this, Lacan immerses the clinic squarely in the acrimony of contemporary knowledge production in order to disrupt the analysand's investment in it. But where the gap in knowledge is more evident in the COVID era, the task is to now find new positions for the same obligation to witness. My conclusion reflects on this, but we shall begin first with the stakes in the matter, namely, on how COVID compels psychoanalysts to reflect on the nature of their practice.

Psychoanalytic ideals

COVID's profound disruptions have compelled questions on how we should think of psychoanalysis's future. Whether it is adjusting from couch to screen to working in the upheaval of mass graves, overcrowded hospitals and collapsing healthcare systems, the sense is that something of psychoanalysis as we know it has been profoundly transformed. For Serge Frisch (2021), the damage runs deep into the very transmission of psychoanalysis:

> [W]e are now coming to terms with the damage incurred to this analytical frame that we had so patiently constructed over the years and then abandoned from one day to the next. We are seeing a disintegration of the rules that analysts have pondered patiently over for decades, then implemented and transmitted to future generations of analysts in training.
>
> (Frisch, 2021, Kindle Loc. 2445 of 5584)

Thus for Howard B. Levine and Ana de Staal, COVID is the occasion to ask more fundamental questions about the form of psychoanalysis itself: 'To what extent is psychoanalysis dependent on its concrete setting? Are the foundations of the framework truly non-negotiable, non-adaptable? On the contrary, is this system susceptible to transposition? But at what price?' (Levine & de Staal, 2021; Kindle Loc. 197 of 5584).

The dilemma is compounded by the absence of a long view. This especially true now, as the initial optimism in vaccines is waning upon news of obstinate variants. Recall the shock and confusion caused by the discovery of new variants which forced countries to wholly re-evaluate their mass vaccination strategies. Social distancing, isolation, sudden lockdowns and long future of frequent booster jabs will be a part of life for the foreseeable future, but only if humanity makes it in time against COVID's morbid efficiency. The consensus now is that vaccination is a defensive option at best but it allows us to at least salvage vestiges of the familiar. Just as one new normal will quickly make way for another, so too will every claim about our post-COVID world be coloured with anxieties of temporariness.

The problem is not so much uncertainty. It is that the uncertainty is punctuated by crises. This is as disruptive as opposed to stabilising uncertainty, one that leaves us in constant unrest. If what we can or cannot know is subject to the jagged waves of this disruption, then psychoanalysts must operate in a world whose shape is constantly changing. But the problem is not practical. It also has much to do with the current state of knowing and knowledge. The daily inundation of information leaves us constantly suspicious over what is actually true, in a process that makes us in turn more dependent on various authorities of knowledge. But it doesn't help that the authorities too are fractured. The global uniformity of science is harder to sustain as different countries prefer to assert 'their own science'. It goes without saying that the state of emergency we have had to live with makes objective assessment of the situation difficult even with the information that is there:

> The issue with Covid-19 is not that the science is unusually uncertain, but that it is being developed in the public eye and at speed, with theories tested in real time and with direct effect on people's lives. The danger is that when science is presented as a security blanket to protect against the terrifying uncertainty of a global pandemic, people will feel let down when the reality is different, and conclude that science is no more reliable an authority than anything else.
>
> (Meek, n.d.)

This casts speculations about what we should or shouldn't do in an awkward light because it assumes that psychoanalysis is somehow above these divides. Claims about 'the essence of psychoanalysis, on the definition and preservation of psychoanalytic identity' inevitably place the field in the transcendent, actually impossible, position of being beyond the crisis (Frisch, 2021, Kindle Loc. 2590 of 5584). The truth is the unknown is just too great.

Lacan and crisis

It so happens that crisis informs Lacanian psychoanalysis. His approach is organised around the notion of 'lack'. This is the void in the inability, distinct to the modern experience of knowledge, to secure moral and epistemic foundations. This void is a dynamic one that forces us to tie who we are to what we can be certain of, and we suffer where uncertainty perturbs our 'identity' or 'self'. Lack is the ontological gap that all at once disturbs and moves the subject – the one for whom knowing matters – to embark on a compelling but futile search for a solution, thereby fuelling his vacillation between doubt and certainty. The civilisational correlate is the cycle of construction and destruction in the incessant dissatisfaction that fuels modern progress. If we are able to speak of any crisis at all, it is because there is a subject who refuses to face lack and is thus unable to stop doubting himself to be certain.

Lacan situates this within a certain picture of history in which lack intensifies as the symbolic order – the discourses of meaning and values that sustain the modern world's seeming stability and meaningfulness – is disintegrating. This in turn leaves us vulnerable to what he calls 'the Real', the force of what had to be repressed in order for the symbolic order to hold. The key turning point was the crisis in the scientific revolution, the Copernican turn that sees man dislodged from the centre of his own cosmology. This forced a gap in knowledge as the existential apprehensions that once found refuge in established metaphysical systems became aimless. But while this is typically narrated as a loss of faith, Lacan is keen to stress its affective strain, as the impossibility of certainty produces a desire for a similarly impossible body.[1] A divorce between word and world dislodges the signifier from any fixed referent and disorganises the drive to divide the subject who must now speak without a viable epistemological compass. Consequently, the clamour for knowledge to overcome this divide becomes an imaginary investment in the ideal of a unified self that will be jarred by a body made anxious by the now limited power of the signifier. The modern ego can 'only live in his own head' or, as Lacan says, 'has no place for others' because the subject's realm of possible meaning is shrinking (Lacan, 2002, p. 31). But this occurs where the value of the subject's words diminishes against the ever-growing disconnect with his corporeality. The symptom 'speaks' where the subject is interrupted by inexplicable pulsations, whose strangeness he embodies as a mysterious burden. Lacan would continue to theorise psychoanalysis through this gap that presses as the signifier tries and fails to pacify the Real. But it is less acknowledged that this is a historical gap, with a spark in an eventual crisis.

This gap is the insight behind Lacan's claim that 'there is cause only in something that doesn't work' (Lacan, 1998, p. 22). The historical rupture suffered by the West made foundations impossible, with the notion of 'cause' thrown into symbolic failure as every attempt to come to grips with the reason how or why stresses an already-deepening ontological malfunction. Every measure to seize the gap and close it can only be provisional before the Real breaks forth, compelling more penetrating and futile attempts at solutions. It is here that scientific capitalism acquires its hegemony. As the 'master discourse' of modernity, it regulates the dynamic of knowledge and exclusion required for civilisation to sustain its semblance of stability. Where capitalism re-organises the world into a realm of exchangeable and accumulable objects, science purifies knowledge for certainty. This semblance of stability cannot hold, of course, as it only amounts to a heightened ebb and flow of consumption and refusal, where breakthroughs are soon questioned and discarded.

The general outline of the Lacanian approach is of course not enough to resolve the question of psychoanalysis's future, but it has the advantage of grounding psychoanalytic work in crisis mode. It accounts for how modernity is a series of traumas that constantly reveals the tenuousness of our symbolic resources. In this sense, COVID is just another moment in the longer series of crises that highlights the urgent need for analysis, a series of crises that also includes the two World Wars, decolonisation, Mutually Assured Destruction, the 2008 global financial crisis and the environmental catastrophe. With this historical view, there is no reason why COVID should be more of a crisis than the Sixth Mass Extinction, unless we were wrongly assuming that there was no crisis worthy of a psychoanalytic wake-up call before COVID. Seen as a worldly practice, embedded in the events that shock and disrupt humanity, crisis is always already the stuff psychoanalysis works with. There were no intervals during which psychoanalysis could assume business as usual, no 'normal' for psychoanalysts to uphold. Thus, if psychoanalysis is to evolve it must be through and not 'against', the crisis. Rather than offer wisdom or solutions for the good life, psychoanalysis is to be attentive to the nature of the breakdown.

The subject is history

In this regard, Lacan anticipates current attempts to historicise psychoanalysis.[2] By showing that it is a product of historical factors characteristic of modernity, psychoanalysis can be made relevant for various extra-clinical social and political concerns relevant to the contemporary era. But to grasp Lacan's point we must go further. The psychoanalytic subject isn't 'constructed' by history as if it is a passive product that just internalises external pressures. It *is* history in that he is bound by the narrative he must construct to make sense of his void. This in fact is how he copes with the opacity of the cause – the mysterious cause of his suffering – which he cannot confront directly and defensively veils in some form of fantasy, be it nostalgia, loss or indignation. It is to resolve this opacity too that he seeks knowledge. By working with the subject, the psychoanalyst is working as it were with the very demand for history, through which it also works through the tensions in the symbolic order that the analysand uses as a buffer from the real.

Thus, while the historical picture Lacan provides explains the context of the subject's suffering, it is not a meta-theory of treatment. Lacan does not appeal to a political or social explanation for the subject's condition, as it suffices for treatment to be guided solely by the analysand's speech. More importantly, by placing the subject at the heart of the analytic process, psychoanalysis is not an applied practice. It doesn't have a template to be 'used' on a person or a situation. It finds its use only in the existence of a subject who, in his tormented fluctuations between doubt and knowledge, must speak. The premise is that the analysand will only be delivered from the weight of his fantasies through his or her own words and not the analyst's. This of course raises the obvious question – pressed often by non-Lacanians and non-psychoanalysts – as to how psychoanalysis could be immersed in the Real of crisis while at the same time retaining an identity. Lacan's answer is that there is no identity. It suffices for as long as it is Freudian, and it is Freudian for as long as the analyst is eventually present to witness the unconscious as the enigma surfacing in the verge of knowledge's failure.

This insistence on a non-identity sounds less fanciful once considered in light of Lacan's more urgent assertion that psychoanalysis is also in crisis. As a discourse that was born in controversy, psychoanalysis cannot be practised as if it is removed from broader Western historical discords of knowledge. Nowhere is this discord more evident than in psychoanalysis's future, which for Lacan is determined in the training of analysts, and more concretely, in how the transference is dealt with. Here Lacan finds a 'crisis of conscience' that is most symptomatic of crisis of knowledge, namely, in debates on whether the analyst could maintain an 'objective' position in the transference (Lacan, 1998, p. 137).

Lacan cites Thomas Szasz, pioneer of critical psychiatry, to agree that there is a dead-end in the way that the transference is framed to ultimately favour the analyst: *'the analyst's view is correct and is considered "reality";* *the patient's view is incorrect, and is considered "transference"'* (Lacan, 1998, p. 137; italics in original). Lacan agrees with Szasz that the transference is an inevitable deception. Lacan, however, disagrees with Szasz that the transference should be clarified through the 'integrity of the analyst' because this assumes that 'the analyst is capable of judging reality and of separating it from illusion' (Lacan, 1998, p. 132). Lacan sees this belief in the capabilities of the analyst's identity as the source of the theoretical confusion besetting psychoanalysis. It leads to a blind alley where the analyst and the analysand only see each other's ego (p. 132). It also casts the entire corpus of analytic theory and research into 'obscurantism', circulating around the idealised and imaginary prospects of healthy 'selves' (p. 127). But rather than seeking a place 'outside' by which it could be judged by an ego that craves integrity, the transference should 'bring out the domain of possible deception' (p. 133). This requires that both the analyst and analysand are immersed where love pivots to enigma as the subject-supposed-to-know is dissolved. This is the pivot that enables the analyst's presence as a witness to the unconscious and is the only form psychoanalysis requires.

Deception and transference

In Lacan, the analysand-analyst dyad is made possible by how there is a subject who seeks a subject-supposed-to-know, the one who should tell the

subject something about the truth of his suffering. To say that this authority is 'supposed' takes us to what Lacan intends with the concept, namely,
that the analyst's authority, however compelling, is merely imaginary. It
should be assumed only insofar as it keeps the analysand in the session. To
say that the subject-supposed-to-know is imaginary, however, is not to say
that he is only instrumental or that the analysand is being 'tricked'. While
the analysand's choice of the analyst is projective, it sets the analysand on a
course to seek something beyond the imaginary, as he also expects to identify with the knowledge about him that this authority figure will produce.
This makes the clinical situation less about 'wisdom' than it is about the
mystery in the analysand's history, the history he hopes to come to terms
with by recounting it to the analyst. The subject-supposed-to-know is thus
not about keeping the analysand talking. It is also about moving him closer
to the enigma of his being, the enigma out of which we will hear something
of the unconscious.

This takes us to Lacan's definition of transference. It is not just anything
the analysand feels for the analyst. Transference enables a certain structure
with which the clinic can work through the analysand's unconscious. It is
to be used as an opening that avails the analysand to a deeper investment
in the analyst's inquiries and provocations. The analyst should therefore
refrain from providing the analysand advice or meaning and pay attention
instead to the analysand's signifiers. He questions the analysand's timing
and choice of words, pointing out notable slips, figures of speech and metaphors for what the analysand might say about them. The analyst listens not
in some spirit of objectivity or neutrality but to gradually defamiliarise the
analysand from his own speech. If the analysand veers towards closure and
clarity, the analyst keeps the process open by continuously directing the
analyst to reflect on what he says and how.

As the process continues, the subject-supposed-to-know becomes more
than simply a practical necessity for the sessions. As the locus of the analysand's enigma rather than a 'personality', the analyst stands in for the
analysand's Other, that is to say, the unconscious source of the analysand's
speech. By speaking of his travails and past to the analyst, the analysand is
effectively externalising his lack, 'handing it over' to 'the field of the Other',
with the hopes that the analyst will enlighten it (Lacan, 1998, p. 188). Consequently, the end of analysis should see this situation inverted by which the
analysand embodies his lack. Where lack was previously 'concealed' and
transposed onto the subject-supposed-to-know, the analyst should eventually realise that no such person or object was needed to begin with, the realisation that stages the belated 'afterwardness' of the unconscious encounter.
The subject-supposed-to-know is thereby 'liquidated:' his knowledge or
expertise is revealed for its fictitious quality, as the basis for the narrative
the analyst constructs and wishes to overcome (Lacan, 1998, p. 267). The
mystery is no longer in the clinical dyad, or the object of the analysand's
narratives, but is re-affected in the analysand. Lacan's rather disparaging

descriptions of analyst's imaginary authority – as clowns and effigies – assume the importance of this eventuality.

The rather schematic way I have described this process belies how it is moved by a *demand* for love, the lack that persists in spite and because of love. In a sense this just refers to the existential nothingness that seeks completion, but it is 'love' in a more familiar sense in that this search for completion is organised around certain objectal images and fantasies that endure due to the particularity of the analysand's history. This accounts for the analysand's investment in the figure of the analyst, and consequently the deceptive nature of the transference. It is deceptive insofar as the analyst at some level is convinced – and as a tall order it is a narcissistic conviction – that fulfilment is not impossible. Love from the analyst's side is in handling this demand delicately, reeling it into the session to be eventually estranged. Indeed, the analyst is liquidated in this spirit, to ensure that the sessions are more attentive to the analysand's demand for love than they are about analytic authority. Given that the analyst's aura is implicated in the demand, it is dissolved where the analyst, so situated in the analysand's speech, can no longer naively 'use' the rules, theories and concepts that had guided him the entire time. This is what Lacan means when he says that the unconscious is on the other side of love. Love is the ruse that must be traversed and overcome, by analyst and analysand alike, for lack to be embodied: 'what is there, behind the love known as transference, is the affirmation of the link between the desire of the analyst and the desire of the patient' (Lacan, 1998, p. 254).

The liquidation of the transference then is not about the analyst's professional integrity. It emerges out of the mess where the transference is met, as a chance event where knowledge and clarity were initially sought. It is difficult enough, as Roberto Harari (2004) stresses, that the transference sees the analyst become the slave, as his mastery of the situation, as the repository of knowledge, is tested by the analysand persistently asking why. The analyst's desire consequently is tasked with a delicate responsibility of handling the demand for love, where the judgements and imprints of his own historical relationship with love must be refused. It comes down to his resolve by this point: 'The analyst's desire is not a pure desire. It is a desire to obtain absolute difference. . . . There only may the signification of a limitless love emerge, because it is outside the limits of the law, where alone it may live' (Lacan, 1998, p. 276). And it is out of his successful handling of this difference, to witness difference as it surfaces rather than to be neutralised into concepts and meaning, that the analyst himself can love.

In this regard, the liquidation of the transference, where the analyst comes to lack, is also the condition for the analyst's freedom:

> [T]he subject is subject only from being subjected to the field of the Other . . . That is why he must get out, get himself out, and in the getting-himself-out, in the end, he will know that the real Other has,

just as much as himself to get himself Out, to pull himself free. It is here that the need for good faith becomes imperative, a good faith based on the certainty that the same implication of difficulty in relation to the ways of desire is also in the Other.

(Lacan, 1998, p. 188)

Handling the transference is not a service the analyst offers to the analysand. It is rather where their imaginaries are mutually entangled, where the analyst's identity is also at stake. The transference takes both analyst and analysand from a love that refuses lack to one that sees lack as its condition.

Revolution

It is noteworthy, however, that Lacan regards this as a matter of psychoanalysis's scientific status, which he calls 'science itself'. Where science is generally understood as the study of nature, science itself is the radical inquiry into the very basis of certainty. Where science extracts knowledge from a taken-for-granted world of objects, science itself is about the grounds on which we can know at all. The former merely denies the gap in knowledge, but the latter is situated in the contradictions of this gap. Lacan makes this distinction to explain psychoanalysis's revolutionary quality: it was discovered where science couldn't come to grips with the unconscious, where it faced the point at which its object of knowledge has no grounds for certainty. This distinction, to be sure, is not methodological but historical. Science itself is the historical horizon in which psychoanalytic practice is situated:

> The science in which we are caught up, which forms the context of the action of all of us in the time in which we are living, and which the psychoanalyst himself cannot escape, because it forms part of his conditions too, is Science *itself*.
>
> (Lacan, 1998, p. 231 italics in original)

We are more able to understand the paradoxical mode of science itself in how Lacan turns to the sixteenth-century French philosopher René Descartes as a template. Descartes' meditations, as is well known, are spurred by a deep discontent with what he knows, a discontent that launches his probe into the fundamental conditions of his certainty. To do so he doubts everything to the point where his existence is only certain insofar as he is a thinking being. This leads us to the well-known Cartesian 'cogito', encapsulated famously as 'I think, therefore I am'. But what interests Lacan is that Descartes does not stop there. He even doubts the veracity of his conclusion. Ultimately, he postulates that the only way he can be certain of anything is that there exists a God who does not deceive, a voluntarist God who guarantees the truth. Lacan takes this to be indicative of the subject of the scientific era who doubts everything except an authority of knowledge in the final instance. In doing so he puts the truth in a 'beyond', in the field of the Other. Key is how the revolutionary gesture that immediately preceded this conclusion – where the 'I am' is located at the lack in the flow of doubt and 'doubt is recognised as certainty' – is eventually concealed by the need for God's guarantee (Lacan, 1998, p. 126). The Real 'I' is thereby obscured in the 'handing back of truth into the hands of the Other' (Lacan, 1998, p. 36).

The Cartesian trajectory of suspicion is a template of the analysand's paranoia as he comes to the clinic probing the subject-supposed-to-know for answers. But in tracing the formal outlines of the modern analysand, the Cartesian recourse to the Other also speaks to how psychoanalysis should sustain its revolutionary scientific distinction. Where Einstein, Planck and Newton were ultimately cosmological – their purportedly breakthrough findings inevitably evoke God, as an epistemic foundation to explain the limits of knowledge – psychoanalysis is 'a-cosmological' (Lacan, 1998, p. 127). Rather than an authority in the final instance, or an organisational structure or identity, psychoanalysis is to only inhabit lack. Thus, where Lacan does define the unconscious, it is to stress its indeterminate quality, as unrealised, placed in shades, temporal pulsations. The analyst witnesses it in the fissures and cracks of knowledge rather than a hidden substance that has to be brought to light: 'it is not in this dialectic between the surface and that which is beyond that things are suspended. For my part, I set out from the fact that there is something that establishes a fracture, a bi-partition, a splitting of the being to which the being accommodates itself, even in the natural world' (Lacan, 1998, p. 106).

Witnessing COVID

Psychoanalysis's scientific status has polarised opinions for over a century, and it is not my intention to address it in this small essay. It suffices for us to see the particular subject that Lacan believes an information-obsessed world will produce and how psychoanalysis should be positioned in it. For what the analyst also witnesses in his chance dissolution is psychoanalysis's out-of-placeness. The theory fades but also take us somewhere else, beyond the entanglements of the clinic that the analyst is supposed to resolve. It is here in this unexpected somewhere else-ness that psychoanalysis finds its distinction:

> Paradoxically, the difference which will most surely guarantee the survival of Freud's field, is that the Freudian field is a field which, of its nature, is lost. It is here that the presence of the psycho-analyst as witness of this loss, is irreducible.
>
> (Lacan, 1998, p. 127)

Consequently, Lacan's anti-institutional fervour should be understood in this light, that is to say, in the spirit of alertness to the fact that the modern world will always see knowledge in crisis. Far from being a maverick or non-conformist impulse, it is an affinity to how the discovery of the unconscious allows us to see that historical fact. Freud was not revolutionary because he found a new science but because he compelled the possibility that there could be a study of science's historical limits, if one may put it that way. This is what the analyst witnesses.

To witness limits, shades and fissures is to also witness psychoanalysis's fundamental precarity. Thus, while Lacan insists that he is not proffering universal solutions, as he theorises primarily out of his direct experiences, the point he stresses ultimately is not a libertarian one. As witness to lack, the analyst is not to do whatever he wants but to attest to psychoanalysis's contingency. If psychoanalysis is not bound to a form, it is not because it has 'individual freedom' at heart but to ensure how analysts should persist to encounter lack in its profundity, namely, as a state of exception in ways that theories, canons and ideals cannot instruct. If we can adapt it is precisely to be more attentive to this 'medial chance status' of the discourse of the unconscious:

> [P]sycho-analysis is not a religion. It proceeds from the same status as Science itself. It is engaged in the central lack in which the subject experiences himself as desire. It even has a medial chance status in the gap opened up at the centre of the dialectic of the subject and the Other. It has nothing to forget, for it implies no recognition of any substance on which it claims to operate, even that of sexuality.
>
> (Lacan, 1998, pp. 265–266)

I began this chapter to describe the analytic imperative of witnessing lost speech in the engulfing COVID emergency, especially as speech no longer appears what it used to be. Joachim Küchenhoff found that 'Most patients felt speechless, many explicitly stated that they lacked words' (Küchenhoff, 2021, p. 151). He takes the task now to be about cultivating a new kind of listening, where signifiers may not be found where they are usually expected:

> Only we must remain aware that in the Corona crisis it is not just a matter of continuing work as usual in the midst of the uncanny threats, but also of allowing horror and suffering to become eloquent, and that means admitting and allowing wordlessness, even sharing it with the patients.
>
> (Küchenhoff, 2021, pp. 156–157)

Similarly for Glenn Strubbe (2020) the challenge becomes about how to listen to isolation, to find speech in our common distanced humanity: 'we are clearly connected in loneliness, and perhaps this is also what this crisis invites us to.'

It is not as if video analysis resolves this problem. Nestor Braunstein reminds us to expect analysands who are hesitant to speak freely where they are right to realise that they are 'under the possible gaze, and yet impossible to prove nor to stop, of that Other, the guard or sentinel' (Braunstein, 2021, p. 115). In other words, we have good reasons to be speechless. René Lew refuses video analysis on this basis. Nothing runs more contrary to the clinic than subjecting one's speech to the algorithmic screen, scientific capitalism's highest achievement: 'psychoanalysts must refuse screens, because their name spells out the truth very clearly: machines put up a screen, and speech (from the Divine Word to the human word) does not accept being machined, that is . . . becoming an influencing machine' (Lew, 2021, p. 121).

This is to say little of the global trend of domestic violence proliferating during confinement. Lockdown has revealed the disciplinary politics inherent to the home, concealed or denied for a long time by bourgeois ideals of filial stability. And really there's little that the analyst's video availability can do about this. Frederic Pacaud (2020) calls for analysts to try anyway and salvage whatever vestiges remain of speech: 'Although there is not, in fact, a psychoanalytic session, we intervene with these children and their families to offer a moment when they can put something of what they are going through into words.' Where people are speaking, it is less a question of whether it is willed or unwilled speech than how to collect the fragments. Sonia Chiriaco (2020) describes how working with the COVID-era analysand is about seizing the few occasions where authentic speech emerges:

> In these days of confinement, the session is hence inscribed in the parenthesis of the parenthesis and the mode in which speech takes place is of little importance. Precious moment, in which each analysand, outside of the consulting room, tries to isolate himself in order to be able to speak about the most intimate to his analyst.

We know that free association does not happen instantly and is determined by the layered vicissitudes of the clinical dyad, which in turn depends on the analysand's predispositions to sharing and talking in hope for a cure, however imaginary that hope may be. But the foregoing accounts signal a different set of challenges altogether, for they affect the very basis of psychoanalysis. The possibility and purchase of free association assumes that private space should be a safe space. When this does not exist, the form of psychoanalysis as we have always known it appears unfamiliar. Psychoanalysts, being the scholastic practice as it is, defined by histories of textual transmission, will necessarily have to turn to 'tradition' as a way forward. Or it could think of how the world might change with little regard to psychoanalysis, in which case the question becomes less about ideals than where we should persist as witnesses to emergent enigmas. The COVID madness compelled Nestor Braunstein to proclaim that 'Psychoanalysis, too, will never be the same' (Braunstein, 2021, p. 113). But as a practice in the field of gaps in knowledge, one could also ask if psychoanalysis was ever meant to be the same.

48   *Ahmad Fuad Rahmat*

Notes

1 The full quote is as follows from the paragraph that discusses this: 'the Freudian project has caused the whole world to re-enter us, has definitely put it back in its place, that is to say, in our body, and nowhere else' (Lacan, 1997, p. 92).
2 As examples see the works of Brennan (2002), Khanna (2003), Zaretsky (2005).

References

Braunstein, N. (2021). Psychoanalysis, too, will never be the same. In F. Castrillón & T. Marchevsky (Eds.), *Coronavirus, psychoanalysis, and philosophy*. Routledge.

Brennan, T. (2002). *History after Lacan*. Routledge.

Chiriaco, S. (2020). An open window. *The Lacanian Review Online*. www.amp-nls.org/nls-messager/lacanian-review-online-wherever-it-takes-place/

Frisch, S. (2021). Individual distress, institutional distress. In H. B. Levine & A. de Staal (Eds.), *Psychoanalysis and Covidian life: Common distress, individual experience* (Kindle ed.). Phoenix Publishing House.

Harari, R. (2004). *Lacan's four fundamental concepts of psychoanalysis: An introduction*. The Other Press.

Khanna, R. (2003). *Dark continents: Psychoanalysis and colonialism*. Duke University Press.

Küchenhoff, J. (2021). The pandemic crisis as a crisis of the symbolic order and psychoanalytic work regarding imaginary objects. *International Journal of Applied Psychoanalytic Studies, 18*(2), 149–158.

Lacan, J. (1997). *The Seminar of Jacques Lacan: The ethics of psychoanalysis (Book VII)* (D. Porter, Trans.). W. W. Norton.

Lacan, J. (1998). *The four fundamental concepts of psychoanalysis: The seminar of Jacques Lacan, Book XI* (J.-A. Miller, Trans., A. Sheridan, Ed.). W. W. Norton.

Lacan, J. (2002). *Family complexes in the formation of the individual* (C. Gallagher, Trans.). Lacan in Ireland. www.lacaninireland.com/web/wp-content/uploads/2010/06/FAMILY-COMPLEXES-IN-THE-FORMATION-OF-THE-INDIVIDUAL2.pdf

Levine, H. B., & de Staal, A. (2021). Editor's note. In *Psychoanalysis and Covidian life: Common distress, individual experience* (Kindle ed.). Phoenix Publishing House.

Lew, R. (2021). Politics of the letter: Screened speech is the foreclosure of the littoral of the letter. In F. Castrillón & T. Marchevsky (Eds.), *Coronavirus, psychoanalysis, and philosophy*. Routledge.

Meek, S. (n.d.). *Covid-19: However good the science, you need good politics too*. University of Nottingham. www.nottingham.ac.uk/vision/vision-c19-needs-good-politics-too

Pacaud, F. (2020). Intervention in the time of pandemic. *The Lacanian Review Online*. www.thelacanianreviews.com/intervention-in-the-time-of-pandemic/

Strubbe, G. (2020). Social distancing and Lacan's 'discreet brotherhood.' *Lacanian Review Online*. www.thelacanianreviews.com/social-distancing-and-lacans-discreet-brotherhood/

Zaretsky, E. (2005). *Secrets of the soul: A social and cultural history of psychoanalysis*. Vintage Press.

5 A smothered community dialogue during the pandemic

Jhuma Basak

(This chapter was written during the first phase of the COVID-19 pandemic in India due to the coronavirus, and attempts to chronicle the ghastly time of that period ranging from March 2020 to December 2020 with its residing point in Kolkata.)

Introduction

Quite like the artist's creative process, the psychoanalytic practice is a solitary vocation, nurtured and cherished in their subsequent innovative journeys. Psychoanalysis ruminates that every human being, including the artist and the analyst, maintain an essential existential aloneness throughout their life either alone or being with another. According to Bollas (1989), this fundamental aloneness acts like an immanent shade and anchor to all of one's object relations. Eigen (2009) echoed a 'boundless aloneness' that is inherent to one's basic nature. This 'boundless aloneness' consequentially acts as the reservoir of affect that inculcates solitude (distinct from loneliness), connecting one with others, whether in a relational/emotional capacity or through a medium (like the arts). Perhaps that becomes the task of solitude: to connect the ego to the external world and its objects – all of which further gives a counter meaning to one's subjectivity. However, when this 'boundless', 'fenceless', aloneness is not free enough to traverse in its kinaesthetic motion between the ego and the world, not free to dwell in its fluid flow between one's internal mental representation and the reality outside while returning to its sense of anchor, then it may often fail to instil *solitude* anymore to its sole purpose of connecting and relating with the external world. In such circumstances one perhaps loses all meaning of one's subjectivity as well. That is when solitude may become an enforced incarceration, turning it to loneliness.

The corona period

Mentalization and transience

From the psychoanalytic lens, mentalization implies one's capacity to reflect over one's thoughts and to experience mental states as representations,

DOI: 10.4324/9781003255895-6

integrating affective and cognitive processes that may further help in linking internal and external realities (Fonagy, 2002). Thereby, one creates a continuum of relative coherence in one's thought processes and affect disposition. The consolidation of it possibly depends heavily on the individual's capacity for containing symbolization through the process of mentalization. This has an almost cyclic response of enhancement of intersubjective reflection, deepening one's life experiences. One's external social sensitivity and social intelligence are heightened, as well as prompted in one's own affective reflection. Mentalization helps one to reach out of their possible solipsistic jail of subjectivity and employ solitude to connect with the outer world. A reinforced meaning to one's own subjectivity is brought back. The chief function of mentalization lies in its containing capacity for symbolization. Mentalization thus becomes a unique converging point of thought, reflection, symbolization and containment of affect. It further may act as a catalytic agent in the ego's effort to adaptability, especially at a critical, traumatic locale – as witnessed in the COVID-19 situation, when our inner subjectivity is faced with a harrowing time of death and devastation.

It appears that the site for the role of the analyst lies in this juxtaposition of solitude and mentalization, enabling coexistence of solitary reflection and relatedness through the analytic intervention/interpretation. As Charles Hanly stated in 1990, 'At the core of the being of each person there is a solitude in which he is related to himself. Truth resides in this solitude. . . . The ground of genuine analytic work in the analyst is his attitude of respect for this solitude' (Hanly, 1990, p. 382). What happens to human existence when this solitude itself becomes a state of incarceration by any external agency, as with the coronavirus? The situation of the pandemic had brought about this psychic cage of loneliness where one possibly loses all sense of relatedness with the external reality, other than to *thanatos*, death and suffering, that envelops the immediate environment. Thus, one feels bereft of all subjectivity, and a meaninglessness in life creeps in. It may be a growing reaction to the lockdown situation where one is forced into indoor confinement. The 'home', where one usually yearns to return at the end of a hard day from the cruel outside world, had suddenly turned itself into a cage for us. One is confined and is pining to look outside to taste the window of a carefree life that one once cherished, while awaiting with apprehension its future arrival. Especially in the Indian context, the street has a very significant role to play in its ploy of prompting life. The street has been a symbol of life and home for many, a chaotic symbolic sense of community bonding for most. The COVID lockdown created a sense of visible vacuum, dead emptiness in the streets. The virtual experience is perhaps the closest possible reach to that essence of a carefree, burden-free spirit that a person may search for when an external threat imposes such a curbing impact on human movement, life, its freedom. This is also a time when perhaps there is a surreptitious whisper echoing in our psychic corridors – since the all-encompassing superego, God, cannot protect us anymore from this unique virus, now that there is no more God left for us to turn to, the human warrior is in a solitary warfare in this encounter. This is a fragile state of being, left stranded by the centuries-old guiding force for humankind, 'the omnipotent father' – God – who was meant to protect the helpless child against the 'big bad world', but alas now has lost all contextual relevance. Humankind feels so lost and lonely, more so for the people of a country like India, deeply rooted in religious ideals and beliefs.

At this point, one is reminded of the quality of *transience* in Japanese culture and psychoanalysis, how it attempts to view transience as a dynamic transitional phase from one psychic state to another, from one facet of life to another. This way it assists one to remain in the continuum of the life cycle. The COVID outbreak has brought forth in most obvious light an acute sense of impermanence of life. Transience implies an embedded longing for what one has left behind while at the same time it helps to move ahead in life's journey. It silently assists in object transition, which is a tangible physical movement, while transience is a psychic transformation. In this sense, it concurrently reflects on the past, while a forward movement into the future happens, all in a singular stroke. In Osamu Kitayama's study of the Japanese *Ukiyo-e* paintings ('pictures of the floating world', often found in woodblock prints) one may be able to locate a certain treatment of to-and-fro movement between the two worlds of reality and the abstract macrocosm of life (Kitayama, 1998, 2003). The Eastern understanding of the soul and its metaphysical journey through the two worlds in this very lifetime is the essence of comprehension of the quality of the eternal floating, travelling soul in juxtaposition against the impermanence of life. As a matter of fact, in reference to everyday life in Japanese culture, Kitayama (2003) mentions 'cherry blossoms' as a symbolic cultural object suggesting a two-way transition between life and the land of the dead in this world. Cherry blossoms in the Japanese lexicon symbolically personify the inherent quality of beauty and transience merged together. They appear to bring life and happiness around them, and then gradually fade away over time, only to return again in another time-cycle.

The coronavirus has left a condition where one human being avoids the proximity of another, apprehending a contagious reaction transmitted into the body. How ironic can it be that one has started avoiding human contact – what else is left for human life if not longing for another? Humans are meant to live together in harmony in society – unfortunately the COVID-19 situation breeds such a discord that it has the potential of creating further discrimination within human society. And in India when the country already has a history of such forsaken divides and bigotry in terms of caste, religion, class, ethnicity, gender, the human race is truly under examination of its human values and ethics when confronted with its present testing time of the pandemic. A relook at the migrant displacement undergone during the onset of this pandemic in different states of India has left behind a sense of communal trauma. Acute unkindness by civil society and a lack of strategic intervention by national governance further broaden the binaries of class and caste, urban and rural, rich and poor. The situation has prompted a sad reawakening of the 'uncanny' in us, projecting our own hidden fearful fantasies of the 'other' to further justifiably discriminate existing prejudices in the Indian site. In this way we 'abject', cast out, the unacceptable foreign elements in us, as often seen in the treatment of 'marginalized' groups of women, low caste, homosexuals, minority religious faith and so on. Sudhir Kakar elaborates in his unpublished lecture, 'Fostering Humaneness: Some Reflections' (S. Kakar, personal communication, 15 March 2020) the need to create 'repository of unwanted aspects of the self' while elaborating Vamik Volkan's explanation of the 'reservoir'. Kakar says:

> These reservoirs – Muslims for Hindus, Arabs for Jews, Tibetans for Chinese, and vice versa – are also convenient repositories for subsequent rages and hateful feelings for which no clear-cut addressee is available. Since most of the 'bad' representations arise from a social disapproval of the child's 'animality', as expressed in its aggressivity, dirtiness, and unruly sexuality, it is pre-eminently this animality that a good self, belonging to an amoral community, must disavow and place in the reservoir community.

It became convenient for India to dump this 'animality' of the pandemic on the minority sector of its community, be it the Muslims or migrants or any construction of the 'other' as per convenience.

The invasion of COVID-19 has brought about the angst not only of annihilation of human life itself but equally perhaps of human conscience and character from society that grips humankind in today's India. One of the greatest challenges of such external threats is that it has the potential to rip apart human conscientiousness, its capacity for empathy, compassion, leaving one with only one's own solitary timid self to survive. Sadly, that largely seems to envelop the Indian environment. Given the already predominant consumerist angst in human society at this time of the capital right-wing, the significance of intangible human affective dispositions may require deeper roots for sustenance against the immediately available material conviction. Relationships may be torn apart, bondings may collapse and families may disintegrate, leading to a community left with no binding, mutually supportive benevolent force other than only individualistic existence in society. However, in this very critical time, one ray of hope against this barrage of animosity was the saving grace of members of the student community comprising different universities and colleges. They kept the 'community kitchen' burning for months, taking turns to cook, providing food for hundreds of homeless and migrants across cities and their outskirts. The true exemplary future leaders of a sinking India. Sadly, such unstructured, singular effort against an avalanche of misery and hunger cannot match the overwhelming call of the time. And this is perhaps where psychoanalytic insight may help us, in its own humble capacity, to rescue that anchor within us to stay grounded within community, with human bonding, compassion and generosity, in spite of the current trembling times.

Clinical vignette

Ms Prerna is 22 years of age; she connected for online therapeutic work during the pandemic period (August 2020), residing in another city. So far, my online work had been primarily a process of following up sessions or supportive sessions after direct offline in-person exchange of a fair number of sessions, though only for out-station cases. Considering the unusual condition of the pandemic, I had opened up to taking up direct online work (without any previous in-person meetings; also, not necessarily with interim in-person sessions following the initial take-off; the current situation does not allow such travelling possibilities for consideration as it is) – a new process for me to gradually try and become accustomed to.

Prerna was studying for her graduation in the United States, had been there for about a year and a half, and then had to come back to India to her family due to the sudden outbreak of the pandemic. A very articulate young person who narrated her own symptoms and needs very clearly, she had anxiety issues with growing panic attacks in the last few months. She had tried to deal with it herself for a while but eventually felt that she needed to consult professionally for it. Her parents were not necessarily very favourable to it, did not quite understand the need or urgency of her therapeutic requirement, but also did not actively stop her from reaching out to a professional therapist. Prerna explained clearly that her requirement was temporary, meaning that this interim period that she was 'stuck at home', awaiting anxiously her return to the United States, to 'her world', where if required she would consider taking support from the university counsellor (which would be free of charge – and that was important as she felt guilty of her parents having to pay extra for her therapy added to her education, an undue requirement for them).

Prerna had worked very hard to prove her academic brilliance in her new university in the United States. She made sure that she was looked up to and liked by all her peers – thus, solely focused on her academic performance. All her professors appreciated her academic commitment, readings and results, especially coming to a 'first world' country and holding herself so well. Prerna worked cautiously on having the 'right kind of attitude' for a foreign student to acquire 'right peers', 'right theoretical standings', 'right amount of being cool'. Her popularity with her peers and appreciation from her professors made her want this perfect positioning of herself more and more. She began enjoying this but equally felt apprehensive of losing her hard-earned, precious position among her friends and professors in case she failed in any of the categories of being 'cool' and 'brilliant', an unbeatable combination. Her state of anxiety was building up in the initial year in the United States itself. However, her daily compulsive functional activities to keep up to her goals kept her going. She could deal comfortably with it. She was beginning to get accustomed to her 'edgy' state of being, perhaps even invited that state within herself so that it would unknowingly act as an impetus to drive her to move ahead and help her to thrive. It felt too empty without that 'edgy' state; her anxiety became her 'ambivalent' salient companion.

The sudden pandemic and the resulting lockdown brought Prerna back home to India, bringing to an abrupt halt her psychic flow of energy that shook up her entire composed edgy world in the United States (built so meticulously for the past year and a half). The stillness in time and action unleashed her defences, making daily life and functions almost impossible in her home ground. As if the ego almost needed to invoke that anxious state to stay utilitarian, a familiar functional pattern from past years, yet she was no longer in control of this defensive structure that she had unknowingly constructed. All this led to her experiencing a total sense of collapse. Her present helpless state brought about associations of similar feelings of paralysed nervous states in her childhood when she did everything possible to excel in her studies and extra-curricular activities in school. The family had seemed completely oblivious to her efforts, never uttering any word of appreciation for her achievements. Even when she earned her scholarship to the United States there was no celebration, as if it was a most regular affair. Interestingly there was no negation either. This may often leave one ambiguous, confused about the others' reactions and responses affecting one's own self confidence and certainty, as it happened with Prerna. Thus, when she found so much of appreciation from her professors in her university in the United States, she felt overwhelmed. On the one hand she was extremely happy to finally receive recognition from her superego ideals which she simply loved and craved for, and on the other hand, she was scared of losing that glorious victorious position. All of a sudden with her return home it all felt so 'unreal' – in another time, another land, almost like a 'lie' to her, as she referred often, that will fall flat to shatter her world, her beliefs, her strivings, her accomplishments and her newly found self-worth from her newly found ego ideals. Perhaps her infantile defence mechanism was about to go through a transition, and her overwhelmed ego was not being able to fathom out this unknown new transformation. Intuitively she could perhaps see through her own self-created 'lie', a necessary one perhaps, which was actually her narcissistic defence against her fragile ego, but equally felt the need to get out of it – maybe the ego's inherent urge to grow from its infantile survival mechanism to an evolving actualization of the self.

This brought about more sharing of how her family had never understood her, and their worlds have been so apart. They had no idea who she was, what she was studying, why she was talking to a therapist, what was the cause of her feeling unwell when they provided her with everything and never stopped her from anything that she wanted to do. From childhood she was exposed to a different world when she was sent to an English medium school while none other than her father in the family spoke in English (who was mostly unavailable from the family) – a significant cultural difference and status difference that she had to negotiate with on her own both in school and back at home at another level. This very feeble psychic conflict got rekindled in a much more critical, overt manner when she went to the United States, having to deal with her feelings of helplessness and inferiority in terms of class, country, skin colour, food habits and language. And just about when she found her mechanism of wading through all that, borrowing from her previous familiar defence mechanism (no matter how frail that may be), she had to get back home, fearing the loss of everything that she had built with such cautiousness.

Once back home, the huge disparity of living practices, thought processes and values that she was increasingly experiencing with her family vis-à-vis her brief life in the United States was making the transition from one phase to another rather difficult to steer on her own. Thus reaching out to a therapist was significant at this juncture. It was becoming increasingly difficult for her to contain her 'lost world' in her present reality at her home ground, which seemed so far apart from each other. She had felt the disconnect with her family long back, given her self-exposure against her familial conformity. She was apprehensive about her own autonomous capacity, which was presently collapsing with the given new environmental COVID situation that brought about a confinement within the house. She needed to be reassured of her capacity for mentalization in order to contain the essence of her transient 'lost world' within her, and that she would be able to rebuild her world, her life, once again as time passed (without blindly falling back on her earlier childhood defence pattern). Given the fact that she was already a 'distant' member within her family and having lost her own capacity to counter this larger-than-life pandemic state, her feelings of being alone and helpless to wade through this time prompted an outburst of panic attacks. Her defenceless state needed an external intervention (the therapist) to assist her to mend her ego strength to confront the COVID combat that turned her world upside down.

It was perhaps essential to guide her ego-capacity towards further sublimation where her academic excellence could be seen as a skill, a quality, rather than to be used as a defence that tends to produce counter-feelings of fear and apprehension of loss, giving rise to anxiety. For this Prerna was willing to go through the quality of impermanence in life's trajectory that she symbolically articulated within the safe therapeutic space. It helped her to participate in the larger cycle of time and reinforce the ego's evolutionary scope that was committed in viewing the world, including the pandemic state, as a more comprehensive inclusive partner in the orbit of life's motion.

Everyday creativity

The reservoir of that 'boundless aloneness' perhaps lost all purpose of rearing the quality of solitude that was essentially meant to have led us to a larger relatedness, both abstract and experiential. Not finding that, the human lot grapples with whatever is immediately possible to clasp, be it virtual or material substance (and one has already been a growing witness to societal fragmentation with its increasing all-embracing consumerist culture). In this state, the deeper quest for human innerconnect perhaps loses all its strength to wade against the glitter of material wealth and power, and one may often be left to pledge a solitary struggle with heavy loneliness and meaninglessness in existence. Yet that inner human connect is the sole saving grace against this critical time. Miraculously humankind is relentless, and thus continues to seek resolution both with the object-world and with one's own subjectivity – and creativity may be one such magical element that helps one create that bridge between them to sail through such harrowing times. In this context creation is not about any master stroke as such but rather some simple, small joy of creation in mundane daily existence that may contain the mere possibility of giving us unadulterated joy in knowing that we may still have the autonomy and the ego strength to give external expression to the inner inventive urge against all odds. And that knowledge of one's inner ability to continue this dialogue of life affirmation, *eros* (life drive) in spite of external *thanatos* (death drive), perhaps adds to one's ego strength to act as a reservoir of resilience. The innumerable trials of humdrum in simple creations may hold the probability of echoing similar wonders that a child may have experienced in its earlier phase of life when exploring, experimenting, with anything and everything that it could lay its fingers on, including its own faeces. A certain kind of everyday creation that may gradually become a constant internal companion that continues to nurture the ego like an ever-abundant mother against an external 'all-engulfing' situation of the pandemic.

It is not much of a surprise then to find the virtual world, like Facebook, being flooded with millions sharing their creative ventures, making that unique creative process into a daily prosaic companion to their mundane existence. Be it singing, dancing, cooking, reading, reciting, rapping – all in an attempt to find meaning for that inner subjectivity so that it stays anchored in its daily practice of the life-driven force. Perhaps when a sublimated, abstract relatedness becomes evasive, then one desperately tends to cling to the ground level of existence, makes do with whatever is immediately available. This, however, is not to be disregarded as some mere trivial exhibitionistic exercise. since virtual social media are usually projected to be so, but to be perceived as one's desperate effort for that same subjectivity to find its crux, its meaning, in this moment of impermanence created by a dilapidating time with all its banality.

India

The politics of streets

In this country today's hope lies in its recollection of the repeated survival of its people and humanity through previous horrific environmental and political adversities down centuries – be it the anthropogenic Bengal Famine of 1943, where millions lost their lives due to starvation, malnutrition, unsanitary conditions, malaria, or the Bombay Plague in 1896, when the disease of bubonic plague got carried into the land of Bombay through its sea route by ships coming from other surrounding ports. The anthropogenic 1943 Bengal Famine only adds to the appalling plight of humanity itself *(and in that respect I feel compelled to make this single association, standing at the juncture of a ghastly time of the second wave of the coronavirus in India – April and May 2021 – a frightful, helpless and at the same time an enraging witness of a similar 'man-made disaster' promoted by the sheer negligence of the political leaders of the country, its systemic failure for decades, all crashing together in a national medical catastrophe, aggravating the horrific COVID state within the country).*

The Bombay Plague of 1896 had the city of Bombay drenched with rain and inadequate sewage system, along with its unsanitary human and animal waste, all of which built into the threatening spread of the disease of plague killing millions in the city of Bombay alone. Although the two calamities occurred in two different centuries, both hit India during its colonial phase, making the national resistance history more layered, leaving behind its impact of a crumbling state of affairs over decades. Yet it regained its socio-economic status along with its human concerns over time. Both situations amounted to a huge population displacement, leading to catastrophic disruption of the social fabric in India. But phenomenal achievements of the human race nursed society back to rebuild itself into a healthy structured edifice once more, as well as reclaiming its momentarily lost human compassion for the race. The coronavirus pandemic is possibly the most informed, documented, tracked human cataclysm witnessed in the post-modern era. Thus it gives one a structural and progressive strategy in order to combat this invisible invader of the entire human race – at least that is the hope.

One has, however, also witnessed how often human frailty stands bare in the hands of nature, as seen during Cyclone Amphan, which hit the city of Kolkata on 20 May 2020. A most shattering experience in the last hundred years for the people of West Bengal and the city of Kolkata (the metropolitan city of the east in India), it added to the already wrecked dream of life by the COVID outbreak. Amphan left millions uprooted with no electricity, water or food for days and weeks, nor telecommunication, the city ransacked off all its trees which had stood ground for decades, shielding its scorched soil of history. One wonders how many more decades it will take to rebuild this city's functional, living system, leave aside the trees that were the only sign of warmth, serenity, beauty for this parched metropolitan city projecting a painful sight of a historical loot and decadence. In spite of such well-informed tracking of the cyclone, it failed to prepare the city and the human mind from collapsing with all its vulnerability, adding to the degeneration in the environment caused by the coronavirus. The joint impact of the coronavirus and the Amphan has had a desolating imprint on the streets of Kolkata.

The streets of this city are not mere roads for commuting but have been the hub of community life itself, social exchange and connect across caste and class, homes for innumerable, including the site for woman's struggle for her rightful assertion in public domain. The streets have been the site of rebellion and revolution, bringing in all kinds of progressive changes in women's life in society. Women's plight in this country has been critical all along. On the one hand, she had to fight against her own family to go beyond her domestic, cultural, wall of conformity; on the other hand, she had to fight for her own safety in public places. Claiming her presence in the public, she stands to lose familial empathy and thus finds herself alone to fight for her safety in public space. Society feels complacent on the lesson learnt by women who 'transgress' (like the Sitas of India when they step beyond their protective territory of the 'Lakshman Rekha' of their familial walls). The pandemic has brought about a shooting rise in domestic violence, making it critical for women to stay safe indoors. On 24th March 2020 the prime minister of India formally announced a nationwide lockdown due to the coronavirus. Within a fortnight's time the National Commission of Women in India reported a 100 per cent rise in complaints of domestic violence cases in the country. As for the public domain for women in India, it is increasingly getting unsafe with an ever-increasing public assault and violence against women. According to the National Crime Records Bureau of India, there is a record of 88 rape cases per day in 2019 – a doubling of the number of rape cases in the last 17 years (Rai, 2019). So, where is the realm for women in India that she is safe or free to reside, that she claims to be her own?

Streets are the essence of life in India, chaotic and ambivalent in character. In other words, the historically chaotic streets of India have been with its strange sense of violence, outcry, justice, celebration, a home and life for its people. It has helped them to stay anchored to the spirit of life-driven force, given them an unusual sense of order in existence. With its assault by the virus and the cyclone, this impression of an extraordinary sense of ambivalent life in the streets of Kolkata/India got disrupted, leaving the dwellers abandoned awaiting their claim over the streets for life. The injunction of curfew in many of the states during the pandemic charged in 2020 unfortunately awaits lifting – one wonders if it is equally applicable when political rallies favouring different political parties and their leaders overrule the decree; or, is it just kept to exercise legal prohibitions against civil movements fighting injustice and unfair practices by ruling and governing agencies of the country? Is this yet another systematic isolating process, cast in the guise of this pandemic time, used to its advantage by the political parties, the state, to divide and rule humankind?

Kakar elaborated, 'recognition of the nature of human reality – namely, that each one of us is deeply embedded with other human beings as also connected to animate and inanimate nature, an order that is only kept from breaking down by humanness'. Along similar lines, perhaps the streets resonate to be an extension of that 'inanimate nature' for the people of India, making it so vital to be studied to understand its people and their angst for life. The spiritual philosophy of India is embodied in the thoughts of the great mystic poets of the country, namely, Kabir, Tukaram and Mirabai, whose songs were meant to be sung and danced in the streets, breaking all barriers of class, caste and gender, seeking an ethereal connection for their soul. All vibrate qualities of empathy and kindness as binding forces towards humanness that joins grounds in the streets of the country, of life.

Consciousness – an objective-cognitive and subjective-affective pathway

This virus inquisitor, unfortunately, has equally rummaged other structural schemas in society too which had so far acted as significant external pillars of agency in constructing the individual's internal psychic framework, its capacity for containment and symbolization in life. Such societal structural schemas have had a subsequent impact of imparting self-composure and equanimity in an individual's growth as maybe desired from a mature adult citizen of a country. For example, the cultural and social life of a region/country, its religious architecture and its educational towers are some such significant social blueprints. Regrettably, political enforcements of this country have often unduly taken advantage of situational cataclysm, as may be observed even in the present bearings of the COVID situation, for their own immediate benefit in terms of exercising power and autocracy. One may recall the history of the 'man-made' famine of Bengal in 1943, reflecting the ploy of the British rulers and the zamindari system of India combining forces to coerce money and life out of the peasants and common people of India. In this perspective, one is intrigued to inspect the current tactics used by ruling political powers in India, who are propagandizing rationalized, totalitarian application of similar covert measures to reshuffle certain basic educational foundations by eliminating primary subjects that are engaged with human critical thinking. Such analytical spectrum further shapes a society's sense of emancipation and equanimity. So, when on 9th July 2020 *The Telegraph*, an English daily from Kolkata, read, '*Pandemic excuse to sterilise syllabus*', elaborating on the various subjects that have been deleted from high school syllabus (Classes XI & XII), it left one feeling dismayed at what petty pretext could there be to wash clean such subjects of social sciences like, democracy and diversity; gender, religion and caste; understanding partition; peasants, zamindars and the state; federalism, citizenship and nationalism. All this promotes and builds an individual's 'higher order thinking' exercising critical thinking, all of which further adds up to one's capacity to relate to abstraction, symbolic comprehension of ideologies, thoughts, cultural and political values and differences. In this country where one's constitutional right to education is still a humungous struggle for an individual, especially the girl child, the cultivation of 'higher order thinking' is as it is very challenged, unreachable, distant, for the common citizen (that which only belongs to the elite of society). As fair governance of a country implies benevolence to its citizens, one expects that every citizen may gradually claim their right to 'higher education', going beyond the 'literacy programme' that gets increasingly propagated under the guise of the present education system.

The enhancement of such cognitive faculties in conjunction with complementary emotional propensity helps in creating the mental structure of an evolving vast consciousness in a person. This assists to contain, govern, act in life in its trajectory of many conflictual and critical moments, both at an individual level and at a community level. It is in this context that the psychoanalytic lens plays its role in deciphering how these various aspects contribute in the development of an individual's consciousness, leading to a collective consciousness of the community. If this holistic development of an individual is disrupted at its foundational level itself, then what kind of ethical edifice is being offered for the future youth of India expected to make choices that are benevolent, generative, conscientious, equanimous for one's own self, the community and the country. And without these qualities how will the youth of this era aspire for the abstract cultivation of the self that may further connect them to the higher faculties of human consciousness? Without these holding abilities how will the individual retain its internal mental composure when faced with ground-shaking tests of life, like the present pandemic (*the harrowing present reality of death and devastation all around from the second wave of the coronavirus in India – a disastrous consequence of an unforgivable human apathy*)?

India's concern for the mental health of its youth, common people, should take a relook to redefine such societal structural schemas that constitute individual human character that affects community in totality. Besides, when there is already a very recent history of massive disruption of Indian universities' academic deliberations, along with its huge student community being thwarted by political governance of the country and the state (December 2019), how can this be taken as only a 'benign' measure by the dominant ideologue as a gesture of support towards 'students' stress' reaction in this rather cynical time of the pandemic? Is reductionism an answer to a complex course of time? Or is it a strategic ploy to create participatory suppression of 'higher order thinking' of a country's youth so that the status quo is never challenged and the caste-class divide continues to broaden even at the level of basic educational rights? Perhaps the existing huge population and unemployment in the country requires a skill-development-oriented system of education that targets job-seeking goals, but does it not have to equally complement a critical 'higher order of thinking'? How will our next generation have the internal resilience to combat emotional volatility against the current and future all-engulfing dangers of life? It needs this unified vision of equanimity imprinted in the joint learning of the intellect in cognitive development along with affective subjective refinement.

Perhaps Bengal may reminisce about Rabindranath Tagore's philosophy of education that incorporated the practice of the fine arts, like music, painting, dance, theatre along with academic deliberations when he founded Visva-Bharati University in 1921. All of that was with the intention to develop the finer, sensitive, aesthetic nuances of human growth that further indirectly complemented the cognitive augmentation of intellectual potential. For the individual, from its very tender growing period, the effort was to carve out an internal mental sensuous process that would prompt one to relate to the inner self, its subjectivity, and resonate its rippling effect to the abstract vast macrocosm (an attempt to nurture the *parole* of the pre-oedipal) – through the poetic creations of music and the arts, nurturing the ground for a cultural consciousness. Tagore (1922) described a certain 'transcendent unconscious' that was located in the deepest layer of the mind which was beyond the location of the biological and individual historical unconscious. The artist was like the mortal man with an immortal soul who had the key to that 'transcendent unconscious'. It holds the capacity to connect with the larger order of the universe, uniting with the consciousness of all existence. This philosophical development leads to the finding of a correlate with the evolutionary human resilience that subsequently acts as the reservoir of sustenance for the ego. An education system that actively engaged in complementing the simultaneous cultivation of the right and the left hemispheres of the brain. The abstract notion of the mind, its impassioned nuances, was equally incorporated into a structure that was imparting articulation, academics, education, applying direct cognitive faculties of the brain. Here, one is reminded of Arieti's (1976) elaboration of 'magic synthesis', where he talked about the artist's attempt to integrate the precognitive with logical processes, in other words, integrate 'polarized tendencies', to give rise to the emerging new consciousness.

Women

Baffled by the systemic stunted evolution of the state, the individual's internal psychic reservation may turn out to be even more lonely and disconcerting during a critically shaking time. Unfortunately, these patterns of systematic annihilation of internal subjective pillars of growth have been executed over women for decades in India. A woman in India is still mostly left with no societal structural schematic support nor with any external individual affective bestower – she is left alone to battle through her psychic sustenance, to continue striving in life for her residual dreams to find some fruition. She continues to strive both on the domestic front and at the public fore. Most women have not had that opportunity to cultivate their 'boundless aloneness' into solitude. In order to harvest that solitude, one needed to revisit that 'boundless aloneness' *alone*, but where she did have that psychic time to do so when she was bound from birth into relational ties performing various social roles and functions of being a daughter, sister, wife and mother? The last being the paramount-defining-entity for a woman in the Indian context. Seldom did she have that metaphysical freedom to taste solitude that gave her the abstract, planetary connection that the self-needed to nourish for its subjective being. The importance of the essence of solitude for creativity gets thwarted in the narratives of survival struggles of women in India. An attempt to comprehend the enigma about women, Erikson (1974) had a significant observation to share about the play of girls, unlike boys, who were engaged with their inner space that resonated an internal fluidity. Thus, from their childhood-games itself women were not anonymous to their essence of solitude as such – their biological formation of the womb, including the many physiological transitions like menstruation, lactation, menopause, may often play an innate role in prompting an intrinsic inner space within their body and mind for birth/creation and innumerable psycho-biological transitions in their life's course, both literally and symbolically. These could ignite a kinaesthetic foundational connection to a rich elemental ground for a generative, innovative potential that had a dynamic flow of continuity. Unfortunately, this potentially rich ground more often just simply got lost for the woman due to the systematic structured and practised, cultural and social disregard for women in general in India, leaving only the glorified stature of motherhood for them to satisfy their creative angst.

In contemporary psychoanalytic investigations, with the shift in focus in the pre-oedipal mother-child bonding from the oedipal triangle, a very significant point of difference was pointed out by Nancy Chodorow in the experience of boys' and girls' capacity to be alone. Critiquing Winnicott's exemplary in *The Capacity to Be Alone*, Nancy Chodorow emphasized that it cannot be assumed for that state to be gender neutral because mothers 'tend to treat infants of different sexes in different ways' (1989). Chodorow argued that during the pre-oedipal phase, due to the mother's deeper maternal identification with her female child (aroused by the strong physical identification) than with her male child, 'the process of separation and individuation are made more difficult for girls' and may subsequently lead to incomplete self-other distinction within the girl child. This feeling of enthralment by the daughter towards the mother may further hinder the capacity for the girl child to internalize the dyad that calls for a certain symbolic capacity for abstract mentalization, which may further create obstacles in her passage to her free and prospective creative trajectory in life.

However, it may be explored whether the very lack of it may generate feelings of desire for the same in the individual in later years. And since 'desire is a symbolic expression of the will to transcend limits', as defined by Joan Raphael-Leff (2010), there may be light in what Chodorow suggested – that once when the capacity for solitude has been achieved by the woman, it would then be more stable and robust in nature in complementing any man's parallel of such achievement. Maybe the woman's need to re-create the pre-oedipal sensuous nuances gets played out in her future feminine relational exchanges, quietly paving grounds for that essence of solitude to sow its seeds of innovation. Needless to say, this will definitely not be a very smooth process to initiate for the woman since one of her fundamental obstacles has been, and continues to be, her problematic socio-cultural learning of the taboo in 'desiring' at all – dominantly in the Indian context. Added to this intrapsychic struggle of the woman to negotiate her realm of desire in order to liberate her personality to its full bloom is also the multi-layered socio-cultural and political oppression of women in India that she has to deal with in order to find her voice of freedom. In quite a surreptitious manner, the Indian cultural imagination has tried to fill this lack in the woman by glorifying motherhood, a readily available socio-cultural fantasy-product, the politics of which is being challenged by changing views of the emerging modern women in contemporary India.

The psychoanalytic situation

Resonating the analytic situation and its dyadic exchange, one encounters a coexistence of solitude and relatedness which is simultaneously a shared and a private dialogue between the analyst and the analysand. The analysand narrates about its world with repeated revisits to that 'boundless aloneness', and the analyst and the analysand together cultivate a shared solitude of that abstract relatedness, giving it a meaning in life. For the analyst, it is a process of assimilating paradoxes – engagement and disengagement, solitude and relatedness. The analyst listens to endless stories, churning solitude to find meaning of patients' lives and their own counter transferential meditations in life in general. As mentioned earlier in this chapter, this analytic dyadic exchange gradually helps to carve out that dual flavour of solitude along with mentalization to further extend our sole reflection, and relatedness, both with the external world and with our own inner selves. And as Hanly mentioned, 'truth resides in this solitude . . .'; we may thus arrive at the experiential nuance of this truth in the analytic process, when two unconsciouses meet (that of the analyst and the analysand) that further ignites the process of internalization. And thus, a sense of togetherness gets internalized that was initiated through the cave of solitude in the analytic dyad.

In this present state of the pandemic, how can the analyst be free from a shared communal trauma and anxiety that equally has its shattering impact on the analyst as much as it did on the analysand? This may concurrently bind the analyst-analysand with an external bonding of a joint reality to negotiate together, both striving to combat a much larger-than-life situation, both in an unsaid humble method of life-assertion practices against an unknown force. For the analyst, this silent, shared helplessness with the analysand makes it a unique experience at this particular juncture, of being embodied by the analysand's very submissions of anxiety and agony itself, as if an echoed articulation of the internal angst experienced by the analyst. Almost like a silent gift that transpires from the analysand to the analyst through the mutual engagement of the process itself – perhaps a rare moment of truth that nourishes both against such a calamity. The truth of the analyst as just another human being who may be as fragile as another when against any external threat may be somewhat unsettling for the analysand to begin with. But it may also be the very component that may create a sense of proximity that could bring the analyst closer in density to be able to feel, reach, since its position is no longer on any far-above pedestal as the superego in the analysand's fantasy but rather brought to the ground reality amidst its own land of communal struggles. In that sense the analyst may be a degree less the 'other' in one's fantasy and join the communion of 'us' in this horrific plight of mankind, perhaps bringing in only a momentary triumph in the analysand's psychic pyramid, but surely positing the analytic locus amidst the shared communal voices of struggles and glory of a devastating time.

It is often considered that the conclusion of an analytic trajectory is the ego's transformation of its increasing capacity to love and its capacity for work. Lacan added another significant dimension to it by affirming the need of the individual coming in terms with its utter sense of solitude. Quite like the Shakespearean tragic climate, when there is intense turmoil in the external universe, the internal world may often speculate the stormy hour in solitary rumination. The analytic process helps the unconscious to become conscious, thereby expanding the vastness of one's consciousness, expanding its capacity as a reservoir. The subjective freedom to love, work and play from inner inhibitions is not the only outcome for the autonomous self but equally is it important to complement that with a 'caring individual' (Kakar) engaged in the process of generating empathy and generosity for humankind. The coexistence of the autonomous with the compassionate along with the self and the other integrated within the ego structure. As Kristeva (2020) very rightly stated in view of the current pandemic, 'in this current state of war, it is our innermost selves that we must save'. And this chapter has been in an attempt to engage in saving those 'innermost selves' within us, within me.

References

Arieti, S. (1976). *Creativity: The magic synthesis* (pp. 12, 13). Basic Books.
Bollas, C. (1989). *Forces of destiny: Psychoanalysis and the human idiom*. Free Association.

Chodorow, N. J. (1989). *Feminism and psychoanalytic theory.* Yale University Press.

Eigen, M. (2009). *Flames from the unconscious: Trauma, madness, and faith.* Karnac.

Erikson, E. H. (1974). Womanhood and the inner space. In J. Strouse (Ed.), *Women and analysis* (pp. 291–319). Viking Press.

Fonagy, P. (2002). *Affect regulation, mentalization, and the development of the self.* Routledge.

Hanly, C. (1990). The concept of truth in psychoanalysis. *The International Journal of Psychoanalysis, 71*(3), 375–383.

Kitayama, O. (1998). Transience: Its beauty and danger. *The International Journal of Psychoanalysis, 79*(5), 937–953.

Kitayama, O. (2003). Japanese mothers and children in pictures of the floating world: Sharing the theme of transience. In E. Blum, H. P. Blum, & J. Amati-Mehler (Eds.), *Psychoanalysis and art: The artistic representation of the parent-child relationship* (pp. 289–299). International Universities Press.

Kristeva, J. (2020). 'In the current state of war, it is our most inner selves that we must save.' *European Journal of Psychoanalysis.* Appeared originally in special edition of *L'Arche*, No.681, 'The Day After'. www.journal-psychoanalysis.eu/in-the-current-state-of-war-it-is-our-most-inner-selves-that-we-must-save/

Rai, D. (2019, December 13). Sexual violence pandemic in India. *India Today.* www.indiatoday.in/diu/story/sexual-violence-pandemic-india-rape-cases-doubled-seventeen-years-1628143-2019-12-13

Raphael-Leff, J. (2010). 'Generative identity' and diversity of desire. *Group Analysis, 43*(4), 539–558.

Tagore, R. (1922). *Creative unity.* Macmillan.

6 Breaking down or breaking through? Varying shades and states of psychic lockdown and emergence of some movement within

Namita Bhutani

In March 2020, when the possibility of COVID 2019 coming into our midst was not just something that was happening in other countries but a reality, it created a lot of anxiety in all of us. While in many ways it felt so very suffocating, like being caught in a trap, it also opened up and became an opportunity to actually slow down and be more present with one's thoughts, feelings and experiences. For some, it was like being in an echo chamber with nothing but a sense of one's own bad parts. For others, it threw up earlier feelings of abandonment and rejection at the idea of being all alone, without there being a loving family to immerse one's self in. For many it became quite difficult to be alone; they felt marooned on an island, this island being their own room or house, with fantasies of others being in a home full of love and warmth, something so coveted. They either felt completely overtaken by their own neediness or felt the very opposite: what is the point of all this? One can very well survive on one's own. Here, I write about how this time of limited movement and space resonated differently with different people – a liberating experience, a suffocating and death-like space, a no space, a known space, an abusive space, a bursting space – and how in many ways it forced us to move, to enter the caesura of these difficult experiences which otherwise would have continued to trouble, suffocate but not lead to any consistent working through.

A psychic state of lockdown

Meltzer (1975) talks about various kinds of time – circular, oscillating and linear – and how circumstances which threaten any kind of sameness can be experienced in a form akin to breakdown of surfaces – cracking, tearing, dissolution, on the one hand, and, on the other, a feelings of freezing, numbness, meaninglessness and itching. He speaks about how there is a one-dimensional level of functioning wherein we live within a very simple world or drive patterns (no mind) with no real other. At a two-dimensional level, we form a surface relation to things but here there is a capacity for concern, to take in the other: some space to think but nothing can be kept

DOI: 10.4324/9781003255895-7

inside and so there is a circularity to thinking and to our actions. In the three-dimensional space, on the other hand, objects and self can be experienced as containing spaces with the capacity to take in and hold new experiences. Here the relationship the individual has with the inside of her objects determines her relationship with time. At different times, different levels would be functioning in us.

When we numb our feelings either by momentarily experiencing and then bypassing them or using different ways of minimizing them (a narrowing down of focus as a protective mechanism, Tustin, 1992), what emerges is an experience and a state of being locked out even though there is a sense of pressure being exerted from within, producing cracks and bursts in our psyche (a one-dimensional psyche). There can be different reasons why we do this. It can feel maddening to experience our feelings because they are too loud for our mind's containment function, not having received that kind of a continent container (Meltzer, 1975). As Sufiana put it:

> It's like my mother plays volleyball with my feelings. The minute they go to her, she bounces them back whereas perhaps what I need her to do is to play basketball, take them inside and let them be there for some time before returning them.

Is she talking about her experience of only being bounced around (a circularity of time and space) but not really being held inside by her objects?

Yet, when this hushing happens, it leads to an experience akin to dulling or deadening ourselves, like a horse with blinders who does not fully partake in life and its experiences. It's a minimization of what comes our way in a bid to not take all of it in, as it feels too much. Reality feels too much so it must be hushed up even if it is something that we have wanted for long. It's a wish to remain in an untampered state, as a young woman said, who would rather remain locked up in a fantasy state than engage with her own immediate reality.

Alina Schellekes (2019), in her paper 'Arid Mental Landscapes', remarks:

> The concept of mental void usually refers to a psychic empty area lacking content, form, structure, meaning and symbolic representations, all expressed through images such as abyss, chaos, black hole, emptiness, nothingness, stillness. The evocative power of these images reflects the very nature of the underlying, unbearable anxieties, namely of falling forever, of dissolution into a formless state, of being emptied of one's own psychic existence and thinking abilities, of losing contact with self and other.
>
> (p. 95)

Schellekes mentions Lutenberg's (2009) two states: one, a state of structural mental void where there are no representations, something she describes in the previous quote. The second is an emotional mental void where feelings of emptiness are expressed emotionally; that is, the person is like an empty container waiting to be filled up. Is it a Walter Mitty (from the movie *The Secret Life of Walter Mitty*) state where reality seems unbearable because of always remaining half-formed? Yet, this wish to get away in the form of wanting to go to the mountains or to some other place and to start anew is constantly impinging. As if the possibility of a fuller life cannot be imagined, so this wish to start anew remains a wish for rebirth, a complete overhauling of life as one knows it. This, in some ways, symbolizes the internal sense that this isn't the life that is satisfying. Rebirth fantasies are seen as the psyche's inability to 'bear the time and psychic work needed for growth and development' (Schellekes, 2019, p. 98). It is a half-life or a half-lie as to hear the truth (truth for the mind, food for the body, Bion, 1965, p. 38) becomes so painful that it is constantly touched and discarded in the service of a safer albeit a smaller existence. It is a life where one is constantly talking from behind a glass or one is like a person floating around in the river of life but in a glass bottle, speaking from there, behaving from there.

It could also be a state depicting a kind of a giving up on life, a turning away from it, bypassing desires, longings, ambition and love, as all these feel too fraught with difficulty. Being a bystander to one's own life where 'watching time pass' becomes a way of being. It's a slow suicide, wherein life is lived in its functionality but there is no purpose to it. It could vary between a depressive stupor in its extreme form or a depressive state of lockdown where there is no real passion or aliveness. Tustin (1990) cautions us to be aware of the autistic, hidden or encapsulated parts of the patient's personality which arise because of a precocious sense of separateness from the mother.

The pandemic forced us to come face to face with our realities, having taken away our usual ways of circumventing them. The difficulties that usually exist in our relationships but get suppressed and are not thought about were, this time around, hard to ignore. The restriction on mobility challenged us in very different ways. In the absence of the usual avenues available to us for coping by tuning out our real feelings, we were forced to confront our truth again and again.

From a state of incubation to stepping out

When we don't know how to process our own emotions, it becomes often a game of touch and go or hide and seek. We feel stuck in our own heads unable to make sense of what's going on, often feeling half in and half out. Sadness becomes a sulk where, instead of feeling that there is a receiving or a meaning-making breast, it feels like an inverted nipple has been taken in and is being sucked on; it becomes a state and space of obsessive rumination.

Shubha has been coming to me for many years now. She always starts the session by saying, 'Nothing, there is nothing, blankness', but once she manages to get over her initial anxiety, she has much to say. In fact, when she manages to get close to hearing what is happening inside, she says that there are too many thoughts running in her head and she does not know which one to talk about. She feels extremely stuck, not able to move in her personal or professional life. She comes from a family where women are not supposed to work outside the home, just be good homemakers. That is what she had seen her mother do. There was also a sick mother who seemed to have passed on her sense of suffocation, of having led this cloistered existence, to her daughter. Leaving this space was very difficult. The relationship she got into was one where there were experiences of violence, bloodshed, obsessiveness, which further shunted her back into her home. When we started working, she managed to go out and study, but that spark could not be sustained and she soon went back into this big, beautiful but banished existence. She brought this dream in which a senior person along with another colleague has come to look at her wares and as they touch them, the things start to break. This is the day after she gets a lot of appreciation from her senior, her work being compared to some very unique and inspiring individuals. It's as if her capacity to contain this excitement is challenged and the containers start bursting/leaking. There is no parental permission to actually exhibit her work, to come into herself and to use it for personal growth. It's as though she cannot be allowed to go towards a three-dimensional experience of herself. She brings this other dream in which she is a child and is peeking outside through a glass door. There is a verandah which separates her from the outside gate. Outside the gate, there are bulls running but she can only peek out.

When COVID struck, she found it to be not very difficult. For her, it was not very different from her usual existence as she did not really have much to do with the outside world. Being locked in was a familiar experience for her. However, soon the outside world seemed to be nothing but a replica of her internal world and that became very suffocating. After months of being afraid to step out, she started fearing staying inside locked up in this jail, which until then was just a sanatorium, a place of retreat.

A bomb blast of feelings

This was a time when no one wanted to be alone. Being alone meant facing the possibility of this virus overwhelming our bodies and our minds without there being any supportive other to help us through this, the only thing that could provide any succour at such a time. This woman who had her partner in another city was in a state of despair at not being able to travel to be with him, the only person she would have liked to be with, now that the end of the world was here. Esther Bick (1964) talks about the lack of skin cover and how without that skin, everything is an attack on the body and the mind. It was this skinless psyche that was coming more to the fore during this time of fear and anxiety.

An oobleq of feelings

This image, of an oobleq which is made with water and cornflour, was brought by a patient. When you touch it, it feels fairly solid, but when you push your fingers in it, it becomes all gooey and something you can play with; if you pick it up, it slips through your fingers. She also brought these images of feeling too solid or wanting to be in a bubble bath all the time, and even though she felt now she was more present than ever, there was this fear that she was not able to stay with the moments, they would slip away from her fingers. I realized that on the one hand there was this fear of death, of not knowing what would happen (some very real feelings given the pandemic), while on the other hand there was the wish to remain outside her anxieties, not wanting to enter them. She felt scared that if she entered them, it would feel like death, a falling out into nothingness and how somewhere between the two stood this possibility of being more there, more in touch with her own feelings, playing with them, being with others.

In another moment, that same oobleq could feel like it had elongated and distended to such an extent that it seemed there was no way of escaping it. Her mind felt like it was in a state of overdrive and she could not switch it off. She was not able to sleep and the only way she could manage was by reading some very boring books in a bid to slow it down. What had felt like this great opportunity to be more present now felt suffocating and exhausting.

This bipolarity of experience, especially during the pandemic, was being touched where, on the one hand, there is severity, starvation and harshness and, on the other hand, there is too much abundance and fantasies of magical rescue. A 20-year-old man would starve himself to such an extent that for days he would not eat till his stomach would burn and only then would he do something to assuage this kind of starving hunger. He said he had always been like this. He brings this dream of going to his friend's house with a lot of food, the kind he likes, which he does not get hold of easily, and yet this friend will not open the door to him. I felt that he was talking about a disappearing, inaccessible mother who would not give this baby the love, the nourishment that he needed to feel the fullness in his stomach. Only when he was starving would he be allowed to take in something and this cycle had to be repeated. Along with these rescue fantasies, he experienced deep, unmitigated rage, in which there would be dreams and images of people having accidents, with vehicles going over their faces till there is nothing but pulp (the apparatus to connect to his feelings completely cut off), or there would be fantasies of either cutting himself or a loved one with a knife. There were other dreams of his mother's vehicle falling off the edge of a cliff. In some ways, he was caught up in a time warp where there was nothing but pain and hunger and deep, dark sorrow. A lot of effort had to be put in to get him to come out of it, which in itself felt like an impossible ask. There were also images of living in a filthy room which had nothing but muck or living in a flooded room where the plaster was peeling off the walls while he sat in a corner unable to move, almost like a deaf-blind-mute spectator to all the misery which couldn't be expressed in words.

My heart will give way

For those who were used to being in a locked-down state, this felt like the new normal and there was this repeated sense that while for others it might be difficult, for them it was a familiar state. Simran felt that she could help others cope with it as she knew what it was like. Finally, there was no shame in being herself, with her fears and anxieties, as now those anxieties had some legitimate basis. However, this deep understanding and sense of peace that she held onto as a way of coping during the pandemic soon gave way to so much anxiety that she would feel that she must quarantine herself in a bid to not hear what was going on around her. She would not reach out to me; she would work in a crazy way, even when there was no work. She would work out many times in a day in a bid to not be in touch with her feelings. Yet those cut-off feelings had a way of finding their way inside her. They would come in in the form of an ache or a pain which would completely terrify her. She would feel that her heart was going to burst or that she was having a heart attack. Here was a baby who I felt would time and again go back to being in that incubator where there was only the sound of her heart beating (which she saw as too much anxiety or having a heart attack) with no m(other) to hold this baby. She would absolutely need to be with someone in the room to make her feel she would survive. She would talk about these anxieties taking over but she also insisted that she knew that they could be handled if there was someone, some doctor who could understand her.

Working on Skype or on the phone created its own resonances in therapy. For some it became too anxiety-provoking, creating a sense of the therapist being too faraway, when she could not also be seen. For some, this necessitated face-to-face sessions. At the beginning, it seemed that adjusting to this new mode was needed. However, when the pandemic continued, it appeared that we had to find different ways of strengthening this connection. Otherwise, it would begin to feel faded in some ways, given the lack of the setting of the therapist's clinic. Did it further trigger the 'dead mother complex'?

Schellekes (2019, pp. 96–97) helps us look at the void in many different ways. She talks about how

> Winnicott (1971) viewed the lack of internal object representations that are typical of the psychic void as a result of traumatic experiences, such as prolonged absences of the object at critical phases of development, or strong inconsistencies in parents' behaviour. These traumatic experiences bring about a decathexis of the object that finally results in a fading away of the object representation, making the 'negative' the

only reality. Following Winnicott's ideas, but with a different theoretical twist, Green (1986) connects between the traumatic aspects of the 'dead mother' complex – the experience that 'mother is elsewhere' – and the work of the 'negative' (Green, 1997); that is, the active involvement of the death drive. He assumes that the death drive is based on the assumption of a negative narcissism that aspires to extinction and that is an expression of what he calls the disobjectalizing function, that is, destruction through disinvestment. The disinvestment can ultimately be directed not only towards objects and connections, but also towards the ego itself and all its previous accomplishments, so that the ego becomes 'impoverished, disintegrating to the point of losing its consistency, homogeneity, identity and organization' (Green, 2005, p. 222). To put it in different words, when the psyche is flooded with extreme unthinkable anxieties that are neither connected to nor contained by a represented object, then the disinvestment becomes 'the ultimate defence against unleashing of instinctual chaos' (Green, 2005, p. 222).

I would often feel like a firefighter, dousing one fire after another, sometimes successfully but often just being there. There was this unspoken fear lurking, the fear of the unknown which now had a very legitimate basis. Renato Trachtenberg, in a supervision, spoke about why this time became even more difficult for all of us – we were unable to dream of a sense of continuity. It felt more like a catastrophic experience rather than a transformative one. Bion, in *Transformations*, speaks about change feeling like a crisis when there is a subversion of order or structure of things. It then feels like a disaster; it feels violent almost in a physical way. Even though he is talking in the context of analytically produced breakdowns, perhaps we can look at all change being experienced as catastrophic. The only way to subvert it is if are able to have faith (i.e., have good internal objects) that even in the worst of circumstances, we will be able to make it through, that even as we enter the caesura of an experience, the other shore of which we cannot see, we will not drown. Rather, we must enter it in order to move forward in our lives; otherwise, we will stagnate.

However, when the psyche is unable to 'hallucinate the object', there is a loss of the ability to represent the real object, and then one arrives in the realm of negative hallucination where one is unable to be in touch with reality and objects as they exist, and what they represent (Schellekes, 2019). It is an inability to access even what is there, thus leaving one in a further state of acute aloneness and hopelessness.

Dislodging and dislocating – remaining cut off

In the chapter titled 'Addiction to Near life', Ignes Sodre (2015) talks about Chantering (derived from Betty Joseph's concept of Chuntering), a method of pathological daydreaming in which there is a cutting off of external reality. It becomes a way of remaining within one's own rosy, wish-fulfilling (pathological) fantasies that provide a soothing humming from which one does not really break out.

In many patients, we see this sort of self-protection: they take recourse to this magical fantasy world wherein they don't really engage with anything in a way that can provide some base for movement. The outside reality seems so grimy that they prefer to remain in a shiny, pedicured version of themselves, away from things as they are. It's a method of self-preservation wherein one really does not move outside of this cube of an existence which, if we put our hands out, can feel very prison-like but on the other hand also provide the security of a womb-like space.

My patient would come, session after session, talking about the same thing. Even though it would feel that we were making progress, working through what felt difficult, but in actuality, there would be no movement in her life. She would talk about her tendency to completely lose herself in a film or a serial and how, for many years till they came to an end, they would be her go-to place, where she would exist. So much so that she would develop romantic, soft feelings towards some of the characters. Her real life did not seem very different from the films and serials she had been watching. Even though it seemed like her career and her romantic personal life were being lived out in a very real way, but at the same time, they had a secretive quality to them that could not be opened up to her own self or to the world in general. The sessions also felt like a kind of a 'chuntering', wherein I was also a character in the service of that fantasy, doing therapy, but it seemed I wasn't being perceived as a separate person who she was coming to, to make sense of what was happening in her inner world with a wish to change things. It felt like the sessions were in the service of actually perversely preserving what was a good, soft place. It was an atrophy of the mind's capacity to dream, to actually imagine there is a better life in which one could actually take off and not just imagine a taking off but which felt like a lie when you heard it over and over again.

The lockdown multiplying

The pandemic and the state of lockdown also gave us the sanction to remain in our cut-off worlds. While many had to put in some effort, after the initial enjoyment of this state of oneness between the inside and the outside, after a point it became something that demanded some movement in their lives. They did make some forays in that direction, in terms of finding better work and entering deeper into their relationships. Yet, some others were sent further back into their retreated worlds, with a sense of this state of lockdown multiplying, inside and outside, till there was nothing but this crazy maze-like existence with no way out and no sense that an exit it would be possible even in the future. It was a collapse of any hope, of going from being lodged in a prison to being sent to a place of solitary confinement. Except that in this case, there was no real panic in being left there, but the sense of a joyless existence.

Schellekes (2019, p. 100) observes:

> In various regressive states that are characterized by the structural void or by the black hole phenomenon described above, language and elaborate patterns, structures and rhythms, instead of being internalized as stable representations, are sometimes used hyperbolically as autistic shapes to ward off threatening nothingness. Thus, one can see that where under-structuralization of the ego core is predominant, an over structuralization of its periphery develops, so that an outer rigid shell is formed against one's dread of dissolution (Kumin, 1978).

This is in contrast to states where there has been an internalization of a stable object with a rhythm of safety such that there can be a possibility of separation and differentiation, sleeping and wakefulness, hunger and fullness.

Being in a gully

For others, being left to their own world, while being cut off from outside sustenance, such as coming to the therapist's clinic, felt like they had been shunted back into this horrible, grimy gully. This would either fill them up with panic or there would be some desperate attempts to find a way back into this world, as unhelpful as they may be.

In another instance, an old patient Amaira brings this dream of a cat sitting on her head and going off to sleep. This cat has claws which are like a hen's claws and they are digging into her head. She is absolutely terrified, and when she asks those around her to get the cat off her head, they tell her to not move as the cat's nails will dig further into her head. This is just days after she had emerged from a long breakdown. The breakdown occurred after she was forced to go back, due to the pandemic, to a place she had done everything possible to get away from. She had felt very indebted to me for helping her through the breakdown. However, soon afterwards, in another session, I had felt that something was very odd about her appreciation. In that session, she had been talking about a dog that she had befriended. After listening to her dream, I felt that what she was saying was that her loving parts would soon drop off. They would become doggy-like, licking parts or become her more hateful parts; they had started to perforate her insides, experienced like cat claws, which she also associated with the sharpened claws of fighter cocks which are meant to draw blood. Her feelings in those moments could not be digested and would become abusive, subtly or loudly, either to herself or to another especially, when the setting of our work had changed. The place she had come to for years, several times a week, had gone away only for her to be shunted back to a place from which she drew no nourishment – a place which would flood her, where the walls would have the paint peeling off and she had no way of keeping her head above the waters.

She could not access the therapist's clinic and even though we were still continuing our work online, it felt like a fake connection to her. As a result, it seemed she was stuck in her head, in this big bad world with no way out. This was a place where there was no creativity, no work, only a sense of being controlled by others, not being given what she wanted. I felt that, for her, facing this reality where she was not given access to the world she had held on to, because of the pandemic, was akin to being abused. She would talk about doing things the way others wanted her to, she felt very controlled and she wondered why she should be in that relationship. It felt like she would end up creating these barriers when she feels hurt. Her curiosity, her intellect and her creativity would get stifled and locked out in the process. Either it is that or there are no barriers; it all flows openly. She does not know how to modulate what she is experiencing, without there being any barrier between her inside and outside, her and the other, so she must create these shutters which then end up locking her inside completely.

Conclusion

In this chapter, I have tried to show how this state of mental, emotional lockdown can arrive from different parts in us – a desire to not acknowledge reality, a difficulty or refusal to process what is going on inside and outside, a wish to minimize pain, a giving up of hope and agency. I explore how the pandemic further put us in touch with these core ways of our being. However, it was not all bad because in many ways it forced us to be more immersed in our emotional experiences, helping harness the transformative potential in our relationships with our own desires, ambitions, aspirations, feelings andf thoughts, thereby allowing for some movement in our lives. While therapy on phone/Skype felt faded for some, necessitating face-to-face work, for others, thoughts and anxieties of re-establishing the contact had to be borne such that there was a sense that 'mother is there'.

References

Bick, E. (1964). Notes on infant observation in psycho-analytic training. *International Journal of Psycho-Analysis, 45,* 558–566.

Bion, W. R. (1965). *Transformations.* Tavistock Publications.

Green, A. (1986). The dead mother. In *On private madness.* Hogarth Press.

Green, A. (1997). The intuition of the negative in playing and reality. *International Journal of Psychoanalysis, 78,* 1071–1084.

Green, A. (2005). *Key ideas for a contemporary psychoanalysis.* Routledge.

Kumin, I. M. (1978). Emptiness and its relation to schizoid structure. *International Review of Psychoanalysis, 5,* 207–216.

Lutenberg, J. M. (2009). Mental void and the borderline patient. In A. Green (Ed.), *Resonance of suffering-countertransference in non-neurotic structures*. Karnac.

Meltzer, D. (1975). Dimensionality in mental functioning. In D. Meltzer, J. Bremner, S. Hoxter, D. Weddell, & I. Wittenberg (Eds.), *Explorations in autism: A psychoanalytical study* (pp. 223–238). Clunie Press.

Schellekes, A. (2019). Arid mental landscapes and avid cravings for human contact: Beckettian and analytic narratives. *British Journal of Psychotherapy, 35*(1), 91–106.

Sodre, I. (2015). Addiction to near life: On pathological day-dreaming and the disturbing ambiguity of faking true love. In *Imaginary existences: A psychoanalytic exploration of phantasy, fiction, dream and day dreams* (A. Lemma, General Ed., pp. 232–252). Routledge.

Tustin, F. (1990). *The protective shell in children and adults*. Karnac Books.

Winnicott, D. W. (1971). *Playing and reality*. Tavistock Publications.

7 Between contact and contagion

Sex, shame and the screen

Rashi Kapoor

> *Any disease that is treated as mystery and acutely enough feared will be felt to be morally, if not literally, contagious.*
>
> (Sontag, 1991, p. 6)

The novel coronavirus, as it continues to spread, replicate, mutate and maybe even gain more potency, has brought us very close to the terror of loss. A mass humanitarian destruction, COVID-19, has been a silent apocalypse, bathed in unknowability and finding its way inside our homes. Our breath and breathing has become potentially dangerous for the other, and we cover behind a mask. Sanitisation, social distancing as well as abstinence from contact is the norm to ensure non-contraction, now synonymous with survival. The new code of conduct has absolved us of our most humane: 'touch'. The moment of contact – now the moment of threat, dread, and a painful wait in unknowability – is a constant battle with fear.

The onset and survivability of the virus not only have had its consequences for life and death but have enforced a remodelling of our existence as social and further sexual betransgenerationalings. It has naturally been a psychological catastrophe, which is beyond the scope of this chapter to enumerate. More specifically this chapter will try and assess and enunciate the extent of psychological distress it has had on our notion of intimacy and closeness from a psychoanalytic lens.

Being a carrier of a virus comes with responsibility towards the other that we can infect. The horror of that responsibility brings us close to stigma that is carried by the infected. In the face of that stigma and infection, are we no more than the infection, all of it? Can it wipe out everything else that makes us a person, with our own individuality? Can it disavow us compassion and necessitate a 'stripping off', of love, tenderness and nurturance? Is it a question of the nature of the virus? Or the status we give it? Or how it transfers or is communicated from one person to the other, that affords it its innocence or denouncement? What is shaming and stigmatising about contracting an illness? Do illnesses reveal something deep inside of us? Our own histories and transgenerational histories?

DOI: 10.4324/9781003255895-8

Keeping these questions at the heart of the paper, and with inspiration from my patient's narrative, I try to delicately untangle the complexities invoked in contraction of a virus, HSV-2[1] (herpes) in the backdrop of the ongoing pandemic. The special place of shame in contracting an STI for a woman, in the Indian sub-continent, is an all-encompassing testament on her being and character. Further, its incurability and status as permanent reinforce the testament's claim, besides robbing her of her right to sexual privacy and agency, and further subjecting her to immense shame. Shame encapsulates the unspeakable. It holds a paradox in experience, enlivening and extinguishing at the same time. Agonising and tormenting, it runs through our veins. The ultimate takeover of shame, of the experience of existence of something which consumes and expels us from within ourselves, I echo Eigen's words: 'Shame-am-ham-me-sham. Shame affects you through and through, your am-ness' (Eigen, 2016, p. 62).

The move to virtual work, and the transformation of our clinics to computer screens, led to the possibility of sustained contact, at one end, but also to a distance, at the other. The analytic couch, symbolic of the womb, on which the patient is conceived, is now akin to a petri-dish, far from the love, sweat, smells, motions and nourishment of the couch-womb. Virtual work gave vision a special place, for it brought seeing to the fore as the predominant means to connect. The interrupted gestalt of the clinic brought its own ramifications, but in the context of shame, isolation might have been its verdict.

Using Susan Sontag's idea of illness as metaphor, the chapter discusses our relationship, medical and personal, advent, contraction and eradication of illnesses. Through a clinical case, the chapter revisits the construction of the woman's identity. The clinical material enunciates a re-creation of the lost couch now through a virtual screen, raising issues concerning ramification of vision as predominant means of contact between analyst and patient. A comparison of COVID-19 and HSV-2, in assigning one an infected status, and its consequent implications on the survivability of an individual's sexual self, is elaborated. The subsequent working through of this state is elicited through a psychoanalytic lens.

Contagion and its metaphors: Reading Susan Sontag's illness as metaphor

> *So far as plague still has a future as a metaphor, it is through the ever more familiar notion of the virus . . . old fears with a new dread.*
>
> (Sontag, 1991, p. 155)

Sontag (1991) gives us a very powerful and vivid history of our own semiotic play in unfolding illness and disease. What remains indelible is the individual's fascination with contraction of illness and complementary theorising of the same. Contraction, and its unknowability, has afforded mystery but has been associated with many adjectival denouncements in the absence of its source and host. The individual's intrigue with disease that is fatal didn't drive the need for its discovery alone. It reduced the individual from her status of being human (leper, cancer, TB, syphilitic individual) and inspired a fascination about characteristics that invited such a predisposition.[2]

Disease makes our bodies naked; it exposes us, and in some cases makes our own bodies a source of dread. The modern fascination with personality and characteristic predispositions as testimony to certain diseases gives us an insight into the deeply complex viewing of the person: how the diseased is viewed, and how the diseased views herself. The idea of penalty as disease, and expression as diseases, subsequently changed to disease as an act that could be controlled. Thus, it began to hold status as revealing something singularly about the afflicted. However, syphilis was an exception to this supposed disgrace. It recognisably freed the individual of a personality disposition, but unrecognisably sermonised a personality type (syphilitic personality), 'was someone who had the disease, not someone who was likely to get it. In its role as a scourge, syphilis implied moral judgement about (off-limit sex and prostitution), but not a psychological one' (Sontag, 1991, p. 40).

Disease was viewed as either an instrument of divine wrath or else a form of self-judgement, or self-betrayal. Disease, which was thought to be multi-determined, synonymously mysterious, was considered to have the widest possibilities as metaphors for what is felt to be socially or morally wrong. It is here that I mark my departure from Sontag's wealth of enlisting, for wrath in itself implied a subject position of having committed, to be penalised for. This itself institutes the individual as an agent of her life or an object who must comply in order to uphold that object status. The Indian polis is replete with injunctions where moral is the psychological. Moralistic virtues carried in the Indian terroir are implicated even if not recognised, disavowed or othered in the hope to claim an object of blame and humiliation.

Extending this discussion to the realm of the ongoing pandemic, at one end, and sexually transmitted infections (HSV-2 in particular), on the other, urges a rethinking about illness when seen under moralistic implications when it is multi-determined.[3] Sexually transmitted infections are viewed with horror and repugnance. The carrier of an STI, with moral policing and othering, becomes a receptacle of projections and also subsequent internalisations. The body parts HSV-2 attacks arouse feelings of shame earning the individual an infected status which erotically disqualifies and humiliates, unlike contagion associated with COVID-19.

The horror of death and the horror of shame, are two mutually exclusive experiences in the spectrum of an individual with an infected status. An STI, with its moralistic penance for love, attributed to its least esteemed and carnal version, sex, subjects the individual, not merely to numbers of scientific facts, but renders her as an isolated spectacle for all representations of illness, invoking fantasies of pollution and filth. STIs further, in their non-curability, lose their secret as a one-time occurrence and become an emblem of sexual, social and psychological death. In engaging sexually with others, the carrier becomes an agent, the participant (knowing or unknowing the other's diseased status) becomes deserving of more blame, for it corners the very choice, indulgence, weakness, passion and desire, which are the proponents of study of any cultural discourse.

With modern medicine and the advent of bacteriology and virology, diseases got a new frame of reference, channellising one's efforts to draw causes from effects. Mystification surrounding diseases found its way out when aggressive and fierce methods to eradicate them found its way in. Where does it leave us with diseases and infections that cannot be eradicated?

AIDS brought its own trajectory, horror, blame, and othering. In providing a specific imagery around it, it didn't just remain a metaphor for contamination and mutation. Viruses in contrast to bacteria were accorded a far more complex status. Sontag (1991) writes 'Viruses are not simply agents of infection, contamination. They transport genetic 'information', they transform cells. And they themselves, many of them, evolve' (p. 154). Although hope of evolution and change is characteristic in the nature of a virus, their contraction douses old fears with a new dread. Viruses became bearers of family secrets, being passed along from one generation to another (e.g., HSV-1). They provided a vivid imagery of the body's insides, fluids, blood and stole a certain play from the body, its own fluidity and its play with the other.

A kiss was not a kiss anymore, whose poetic play preserved experiential explorations, but rather a site of danger. Intercourse became an act to be feared, and not just an act of love, in the language it was afforded and safety standards that became prescriptive. This brought about a suffering that degraded, and also gave an identity. It brought a new dimension to illnesses as terrifying, not only because they are lethal but because they are dehumanising. In a misogynistic state, where women are robbed of their sexual subjectivity, making them objects, and sex unplayful (Narayanan, 2014), it only further mutilates a woman with an infected status.

It's an interesting facet, how much our face can reveal about the illnesses we carry. What doesn't damage the face does not arouse the deepest dread, horror or disgust (Sontag, 1991; Balsam, 2008). But our faces are not always a site to reveal the name of an illness. Besides, culturation lays enough significance on the way we look and are meant to hide the sufferings we carry. That which can be seen can become a site for shame and embarrassment. The ongoing pandemic keeps us masked, we are unable to see each other's faces and know little about our suffering. What is hidden behind the mask is not free from our projections, and is a representation of illness itself. In masking our existence, we have lost our very connection as people and have become dehumanised robots, moving at our paces and keeping up with the machinery of life. In coming face to face, one recovers an ethical sociality (Levinas, 1984, as cited in Haq, 2021, Chapter 3), which we no longer are obliged to, for we remain reclused, distanced and away from any socialisation.

Through Sontag's writings one can see a movement in theorising illness from miasmic theories to germ theories and now virology to explain contagion. Now we are determined to find causes and nail down illnesses to their causes and eradicate potential effects. The erasure of mystery and exertion of power through knowledge not only feeds the illusion of our superior existence but also masks the innumerable fears that comprise human existence. The fantasy of eradication is akin to an omnipotent mind state, unable to tolerate its bearings being out of control. An island of its own, the need to eradicate also symbolises the distance it now embodies in the fear we all live in, keeping apart through the ongoing pandemic.

Psychoanalysis offers to preserve the meanings of these miasmas, for they still comprise our very existence and provide a space for exploration, of the many experiences trapped in the living with a virus. 'The couch' remains a safe space, to enable an unfolding of what our control is masking, where our fears can exist, tying themselves down to an illusion that the discovery of a cause can erase its effect altogether. The pain associated with the collective denial has hope in a potential mourning while preserving the singularity of the mourner's experience. Psychoanalysis offers a space to look at diseases as more than just illnesses saturated with distinctly modern evaluations of energy and disaster adding to our paranoia as discoverers, more as agents of a myriad range of experiences in our lives. Additionally, psychoanalysis holds the histories that live inside of us and helps us understand our own journeys, while we unravel our own complexities, irrespective of historical revolutions.

The sex-shame-sexuality matrix

> *Shame functions as both the emissary of the social, a cultural police- person- and as the internalized stain on the subject, flooded with its blush that pulses through the blood, colouring the body, and knowing its sources in the blood of sexuality and the female sexual body. In being born of woman we are bathed in and sustained by life-giving blood; yet it is that blood that inherits the deepest taboos and has infected the women whose monthly shows make life possible and yet must hide their potency in shame.*
>
> (Pollock, 2006, p. 16)

A discussion on sex can omit sexuality, but a discussion on sexuality is not possible with omission of sex. The extremely fascinating question of sex and sexuality is a cornerstone in psychoanalysis. Yet it invokes, theoretically and experientially, a myriad range of feelings; from wanting to banish, deny, disavow, shame, humiliate, yet also to excite, incite and play. Too much of it, too little of it, abstinence from it, indulgence in it, celibacy, promiscuity as statuses rendered to it: psychoanalytical theories have toyed with many ideas around sex and sexuality as a product of psychic life. However, this is not without civilisation's implications on what might be considered an appropriate sexual life. What about an infected sexual status?

Talk about sex can make us intellectually anxious, bodily anxious and also psychically anxious. In ideas perhaps we try to distance ourselves from the real tectonic of sexuality, but ideas have a weight and a body of their own and are castings of the facts they represent. From being domesticated to being split between childhood tenderness and adult passion, to being object-seeking and not pleasure-seeking, sexuality has traversed a journey in psychoanalysis. Sex, not only corporeal but also interpersonal, is not exclusive to the genitals but includes the mouth as a primary site of relatedness (made conceivable through nursing) (Dimen, 2003). Additionally, intrapsychic, interpersonal and cultural determinants engage our understanding on various inscriptions of our desire.

When we talk about sex it is beyond the frame of duality, in a frame of mutuality and relationality, with its messiness and murkiness. Sex and sexuality are about many things, but for the purpose of this paper, I am staying close to experientially one of the most difficult experiences around sex and sexuality, that of shame. The Oxford dictionary defines shame as the feelings of sadness, embarrassment, and guilt that you have when you know that something you have to do is wrong or stupid. I think an essential feature in talking about sex is its 'performative' injunction; the talking of it is akin to the acting of it, and doing of it. But speech in being a declaration is not an action itself, and hence this ambiguity is what makes it erotically, effectively, cognitively and therapeutically powerful (Dimen, 2003; Benjamin & Atlas, 2015). But is sex always shameful?

Freud's three essays on sexuality broke many taboos in asserting that there is no normal adult sexuality. Laden with affection in the move into latency we learn from Freud that society favours and supports the reappearance of sexuality in the boy. This, however, is not the same for the girl, 'the social environment, the cultural frame, immediately captures and stifles it even before it has really burgeoned the sexuality of a girl, introducing a secondary social repression whose instrument is shame' (Pollock, 2006, p. 17). Puberty, which brings so great an expression of libido (in its drive towards discharge) in boys, is marked in girls by a fresh wave of repression. The development of the inhibitions of sexuality (shame, disgust, pity etc.) takes place in little girls earlier and in the face of less resistance than in boys. The tendency to sexual repression seems in general to be greater and takes on a passive form (Freud, 1905/1962, as cited in Pollock, 2006).

Shame, a complex and violent experience which resides in the molecular layers of our bodies, is hard to encapsulate in its voracity, as experienced. Its experience is that which cuts and burns, exiles and banishes, necessitating a hiding – wanting to be swallowed and consumed by something safe (as in the ideal of Sita,[4] being swallowed by Mother Earth – can be dropped

no lower for she is taken into the ground/womb itself, or of complete annihilation – nothing more to destroy anymore?). The seeking is of something
permanent, anything which will keep us away from experiencing shame. It
is what beckons our own invisibility, our desperate need to keep something
secret, so painfully knowing of its existence as to shut down that part of our
existence, split it off, albeit unconsciously – the good, the bad, the forbidden; the pleasurable and the damnable.

It is a calling out, an announcement, a declaration and intention. It puts
the shaming person in the position of power, and for that very acquired
status, denounces the other. An emblem of the outside, always keeping a
check on the theatres of the insides, it generates from relational spheres of a
clash between internal desires and external forces, extending to humiliation,
mortification and embarrassment (Balsam, 2008). The body is the site of
this theatre. It is pulled in to experience what the mind cannot fully capture,
and also, it's the site from where this experience is generated. Some body
parts arouse more shame than other body parts, especially the genitals. This
imposes a hierarchy, pushing the sexed female more into the margins and
as recipient of projections of othering. This othering and gendered trauma
have repercussions for the way women experience themselves and afford
meanings of sexual difference and specificity.

'Sexuality is anything (mostly bodily behaviour) that is forbidden by the
surrounding, especially by disapproving parent who activates the child's
shame. It also creates the excited tension for the forbidden' (Lichtenberg, as
cited in Balsam, 2008, p. 726). From an Indian perspective, a culturally valued virtue of sacrifice, dutifulness, and upholding moral standards (Kakar,
1990, 2012; Kakar & Kakar, 2007) may represent itself in 'people-pleasing',
of a self, depleted of its subjectivity but upholding its object status. In keeping up with these canons, binding and confining, a momentous burden is
also reflective of theatres of an inauthentic self. This inauthentic self could
be understood to be germinating from the pain of shame, hardwired in failures of communication from very early on, in the mother's approving gaze
(in experiments with infants, Tronik et al., 1978, as cited in Mollon, 2005).
Those parts that may not meet the mother's approval are quite literally 'free
for disposal down the toilet'. The mother's disapproval of autoeroticism –
the child's ability to be and pleasure themselves – may also be seen as the
first narcissistic injury. This destroys the infant's body as a source of her
own pleasure and replaces those sensations with the feeling of shame (Mollon, 2005) It is no surprise that the body or sensations arising from the body
also become a source of shame (Alizade, 1999).

To shame someone is to render them invalid. Shame associated with
dependency on social approval becomes an effective response to growing
individual perceptions of flaw or failure, to live up to her own internalised
ideals. Feelings of worthlessness and self-attack seen in women are often
manifestations of hidden shame in relation to sexuality and by-products of a
phallocentric culture (Pollock, 2006). This has particular impetus in a culture

like ours, where there is a collective denial and dissociation of female subjectivity altogether, where melancholia is housed in misogyny. One cannot mourn the loss of what has not been given a place and is denied in the larger rubric of what comprises the Indian cultural context (Narayanan, 2014).

Women have not been permitted their rightful sexual agentic status while enough has been instituted to regulate and control her sexual desires. Similar restrictions are not imposed on the sexed male who might himself be tied down to an all-consuming *enthralling* mother (Kakar, 2003), inciting his anxiety about his status as a man (be it potent and honourable), and what woman must he accept and choose as his wife to marry. His own philandering status remains unquestioned while the woman has to stand testimony, ceremoniously, as pure and deserving of a certain upper-caste Hindu Man. Madhvacharya states that 'adulterous women . . . live in disrepute, contract sexual diseases, and are reborn as female jackals that eat rotting substances' (Vanita, 2005). Not only are there laws instituted to regulate our ways of living but there are those, exclusive to curb and control the woman's desire. The woman's execution of her desire has also carried within it a grotesque image of pollution: 'in my view, to sleep with a woman who is common to many is like playing with a spittoon used by many' (Madhvacharya as cited in Vanita, 2005).

'The fate of an Indian girl's sexuality is a socially enforced progressive renunciation' (Kakar, 2012, p. 103). Robbed of her status as good, she awaits sanctioning and approval in finding quivering words for her choices. She awaits a sentence for exercising her will in the ambit of these established canons. I further imagine an Indian woman's poorly conceived subjectivity, haunted by shame and humiliation, in the wake of being seen as unable to uphold this status. The eyes of Dharma,[5] in its claim to law, only fixates her at her objectively defined position and humiliates any movements which signify difference. This further expels into the margins the woman's sexual subjectivity, when she earns an infected status. Un-couched in the current context of the ongoing pandemic, the eyes of Dharma, of patriarchy, of the analyst in the clinic and one's own internalised eyes become the all-invasive forbidding eyes, an injunction for the emergence of her-self.

'Shame-am-ham-me-sham': The clinical vignette

> *When pain does not arise accidentally but is inflicted as a punishment, the resulting persecution is much more difficult to bear. Suffering then is not simply a confrontation with pain or danger but something imposed with the intention to hurt and ultimately to destroy.*
>
> (Steiner, 2011, p. 7)

Rida[6] has been in ongoing therapy for a few years. Successful in her career, she began therapy in her early 20s, presenting with symptoms of panic, triggered when she was ghosted (abruptly dropped), after being persistently pursued by a potential suitor. Exhausted and very broken, Rida's righteousness and inability to make sense of these experiences left her further feeling injured, humiliated and 'small'. A potent family narrative internalised as a dictum – no pre-marital sex or you will be banished and expelled, as was played out in the story of her 'estranged' aunt, led her to shut down, inaccessible to her own sexual and agentic self. It was as though it didn't exist. And only over the years, in the transference, could this secret unfold.

In the room there was a polite, sincere, dedicated patient; a little girl, re-enacting with me, 'do as Mummy says', where I was Mummy. My approval seemed the most important, as though I did not only bear witness to her suffering but also in breaking down and explaining every action of hers to me, she was relying on my witnessing eyes to testify. The therapy room often seemed like a courtroom, where I was being summoned to pronounce her guilty.

She discovered her sexual self when she began dating for the first time. She would bring to therapy fears about being caught (found out) while having sex or deriving pleasure from any physical intimacy. As a result, she would keep looking for cameras as soon she entered her partner's room. She was being seen all the time by an internalised punitive parental dyad, forbidding the emergence of her sexual self. In the clinic, I became those eyes. Could she undress with me, or would I strip her and leave her exposed and alone, as in her fantasy of what lay ahead in being discovered 'a woman', by her parents? In touch with her father's murderous rage, she'd say, 'He will kill me', and her mother's subservience, 'she'd be too ashamed, and question how she raised me', there was little space for a self to emerge.

Rida found herself to be deeply alone in what she came to retrospectively describe as a non-relationship with her partner. However, she continued to remain dutiful, loving and performing the role of what she internalised was the 'good-girlfriend', taking from the mother who was the 'good-wife and daughter-in law'. These virtues as she had learnt would not fail her. If she earned the status of a disappointing daughter, she could redeem herself in winning approval as a 'good-girlfriend' and 'good-patient'.

The end of the relationship not only marked the erasure of the self but exposed how lost, humiliated and mortified she was in discovering her smallness irrespective of these 'good' guaranteeing coverings. The price she paid for this rejection, and as penance for exercising her sexual self, was a shutdown of that part of her. An object of scourge, she would imagine herself pest-like in the eyes of the other, who desperately wanted to get rid of her. My countertransference would often leave me imagining – Gregor Samsa from Kafka's *Metamorphosis* (1981), an insect-like bug to be put away in a room, denying her any loving affiliation. She internalised this unwant for her as her own insect-like repugnance. Extended to her friendships and dating life this would only be reiterated. Rida's hopelessness and pain in being unwanted would often surface in questions of her insides: 'What is it that they see when they come close to me? It's like they see something and have to run.' What her eyes couldn't see, she believed everyone else's could. Therapy became a quest to discover the source of this un-want and rejection of her. Intimacy and closeness became unimaginable, even between us in sessions.

The final blow of unwantedness came shortly before the onset of the pandemic, when she accidently discovered her diagnosis of herpes (HSV-2). She began to view herself as an infection, of a carrier of something dreadful in her blood (re-invoking the narrative of her estranged aunt). The virus cemented her unwantedness, now with a name and locale, seen by the other's persecuting eyes. The shame was doubled, in being discovered as sexual, and in being a carrier of a sexually transmittable infection. This fear became a validated fact when she was introduced for the purpose of marriage to a potential match, who then revoked his proposal on discovering the diagnosis.

The camera from her partner's bedroom had found its evidence in herpes as a metaphor for her sin at one end, and pleasure at the other. She had been found out. The mask, a metaphor for the condom, with no guarantees of protection from viruses, cemented her repugnance as the object of disgust. Quarantining, initially brought about some respite from the persecuting eyes of the other, now the only visible part of the human face. But eyes also withdraw and avoid contact in the event of shame. This left her trapped and hostage in her parental home/gaze. The safe space of the clinic was also taken away in the move to online work. The screen that separated the two of us was also now our only means to work together. The warmth of the clinic was now replaced by the coldness of her room, while the walls felt porous, leaking her secrets. Shame, dissolving every bit of her, into nothing more than an infection, further metamorphosed her. The assault of the knowledge of a virus living inside of her made it difficult for us to conceive the couch.

Genital herpes presents itself as a cluster of sores, ulcers or blisters erupting on the skin around the genitals. Women are more at risk for contraction than transmission. The infection in itself discriminates, putting women at greater risk. It infects the sexual fantasy with a breakdown of body, the face (concealing, not-revealing), the mouth and genitals (both potential sites of the infection), how to look and what to touch. An intrusive screening fantasy perpetuates which repeatedly summons without purpose, for it has already pronounced its verdict. Rida was asymptomatic.[7] A diagnosis established as result of a blood test symbolised a denouncing evaluation. Her insides lost its repugnant mystery in being found out and seen as herpes. Now, too close to, and trapped in, an 'alienating identification' (Faimberg, 2005), with her estranged aunt, without hope for a future and safety, it felt as though she couldn't access me. As affording her an all-encompassing identity, diagnosing also highlights a poorly conceived subject status of the ill.

'The recognition that being observed can lead to embarrassment, shame, and humiliation allows us to focus on the importance of gaze' (Steiner,

2011, p. 8). The computer screen now became the new set of eyes, through which I would see her (a double-screening). Perhaps I was experienced as 'masked' behind this screen, with my eyes filled with disgust (repetition) for her. Watching out for my own safety, as an authoritative seeing other with power to humiliate her in her fantasy, I too, was terrorised and disgusted. I imagined her imprisoned, for she had been convicted. My eyes seeing her at a safe distance, during our allotted time left her feeling only exposed and cold. I had become the punishing eyes of the other, she viewed me as having, refurbishing her unwantedness and smallness, all of me.

> There is a distance between us, a space I know where I can be dropped. Before I would feel like a monkey hanging around your neck, so you'd at least hold me before I could be dropped. Now there is no dropping because there is no holding. The question of being dropped doesn't arise altogether, because now I can't be touched, let alone be held.

The pain in Rida's words of her potential rejection by my seeing of her insides brought me closer to her need to keep me at a distance. Her infection and contagion couldn't allow my touch, for she felt disgusting to me: avoiding the risk of humiliation was paramount over allowing us a space of connection and compassion. Further, her inability to see me in person, leaving the screen as our only means of contact, also bounced back her projection as disgusting and unwanted, back into herself.

The inability to *tolerate* the otherness of the sexual and its inevitably high level of arousal manifests as the fear of 'too-muchness', both in intimate relations and the transference – a fear that may already be embedded in a specific form of the mother's transmission via the attachment system. This fear is accompanied by a concomitant experience of shame, a fragmenting sense of inadequacy related to the inability to bear excess (the inherent otherness of sexuality), which affects the sense of being a real man or woman (Benjamin & Atlas, 2015). Her love for the other jaded as neediness and vulnerability left her feeling 'too-much', even for me in the transference. This further added to feeling shamed, for being too much warranted her rejection. She had learnt to regulate herself, keeping herself moderated with me, unable to authentically be with me. Was she returning to the script of a 'depressive Sita' (Haq, 2018), or was she splitting – off the agentic part of herself (laws of Manu), or renouncing as penance in hope of redeeming herself (Kakar, 2012). Her narrative echoed a question – how do we feel safe in the intimacy of a new setting, with the reality of an evil, annihilating virus outside and a virus as a symbol of unwantedness and neediness inside?

Conclusion

> *Judith Jordon defines shame as 'affect sense of unworthiness to be in connection, a deep sense of unlovability, with the ongoing awareness of how very*

much one wants to connect with the others' (1989). Further she suggests that shame diminishes the empathic possibility within a relationship. . . . Involving one's whole being in relationship.

(Hartling et al., 2004, p. 2)

Shame can sting, it's where compassion cannot be felt. It is a deeply annihilating experience in itself. It warrants the presence of a gaze, which is looking and piercing inside oneself, and haunts with a sense of blame: '*I did something to deserve this.*' In the context of COVID-19, where our notion of safety thrives in distance from each other, our connection to each other has undergone test and strain. Contact-comfort-connection is now replaced by contact-contagion-contraction.

As psychoanalytical clinicians, we bear witness to our patients' symptoms, which encapsulate in them their individual, family and intergenerational histories. We listen to their symptoms as they emerge in the transference and countertransference matrix, sealed in silences and absences. Rida's is one story of alienated identifications, where her parents function in the framework of a narcissistic regime appropriating her identity (dutiful/performative) for themselves, while unable to acknowledge her independence (sexual/agentic), without hate and subjecting her to their own history of hatred (estranged aunt). She is captive to their intrusion (Faimberg, 2005). Similarly, the field of medicine reveals that viruses transmit from one generation to another. Mutating and evolving, their remnants impact generations ahead of them. However, the fear and dread evoked by the unknowability of a virus, or the extent of its wrath, in the absence of method to eradicate it, is a story of doom. Perhaps our threat to survival is dependent on our fantasy of omnipotence and power to eradicate dreadful diseases. Individuals historically have been questioned and disgraced for contraction of illness. However, psychoanalysis creates room for this very unknowability and the myriad fears associated with the discovery of illness.

Eigen (2016) writes, 'You can't escape an anal reference when you speak of the depths of shame – seeing yourself through your rear end. Asshole shame' (p. 63). There is something shameful about viewing ourselves from not just our behinds but from our genitals. The shame of a vagina, which can embrace, hold and caress, but also feel dangerous for it, can infect in the case of an STI. The vagina thus becomes the space of projections, for all that is unknown, filthy, polluted and all that is destructive yet potent. The patient's narrative highlights the fear of contraction at one end but also pedantic fantasies around purity and virginity at the other, and of the dread of the woman's sexual excesses.

Herpes, a virus that can transmit orally and not just genitally, traverses a distance deep into our psyches. To the eye, is oral herpes less deplorable than genital herpes? Is what is transmitted through the mouth less shaming than that which transfers through genitals? As though in coitus, our bodies and minds don't collapse into one another but only parts, genital parts merge, where one ejaculates and the other contains? Perhaps the epidemiology of herpes reveals the fantasy of sex, which isolates and splits the body, further objectifying and disqualifying creativity and play associated with it.

With the onset of the pandemic, the patient was trapped in an ensuing imprisonment. The analyst, thus, was not only the seeing object (in the backdrop of continuing shame), who in extension to the parental gaze became a repudiating object, but also a screening object, who hid behind a no-contact shield (the computer screen) reminding her of her contagion and repugnance. The virtual couch struggled with a re-creation, for now seeing the upper part of her body and not below the torso was a new phenomenon. A difficult back and forth in finding the right position for the sex we do,[8] the body was split to be screened in sessions. It added to the ensuing fear of bringing into sessions the part of her body that was the cause of such shame, making it invisible to me.

The patient's narrative calls out the cultural stereotyping of the woman's agentic and sexual self. Internalising herself as the object of disgust, where she was robbed of the comfort of touch, gives us the image of a metamorphosed self-state. The most powerful determinant of psychological harm is the character of the traumatic event. Individual personality counts little in the face of overwhelming events (Herman, 2015). I wonder: in the event of trauma, targeted by the persecutory gaze of patriarchy, does the woman take recourse as object and not subject, further perpetuating the imbalance of sexed subjectivity? As though in internalising the man's fear of her sexuality, which can devour, destroy, and even infect, she loses her own sense of self. The gaze holds a special place in how one is not only seen by the other but how one internalises the other's seeing of the self. The eye of Dharma, the one which polices, and enlists a way of life, further mirrors with prohibition, and in effect, to penetrate and now screen her and call out her sin. The cost of pleasure is punishment, and she had to split off that part from herself.

The Indian woman's narcissism is also linked to live to up to ideals which warrant her admiration. Maybe in India we are primed to women without voices, silenced, accommodating, without a past, waiting for a present to be born when chosen by a man. These virtues reiterated by the polis leave little room for her subjectivity. A right to agency then denounces one's status as admirable and also wanted. The echoes, in isolation and quarantine of the patient's experience with first a diagnosis, and then rejection, reiterates her shame as a cultural defect, that repeatedly injures and insults her agency. Medically as well, her sexual agency was reduced to screening and shaming. Rida shares:

> It was the way she questioned me, the gynaecologist, after already taking a run-down on my sexual history. Child, please be honest with me about your sexual history. I could already see she saw me as something promiscuous and cheap. That if I had herpes, means I was necessarily

with multiple people. She just assumed it and wouldn't believe me. And it felt like I needed to prove to her that I wasn't and even if I was?

The patient then is locked into this projected repugnance in a double policing: cultural and medical.

The fate of one's agentic self, attacked in the advent of trauma can make contact untrusting and even humiliating. Between being exposed and crushed at one end and completely devoid of her erotic self at the other, the female-sexed Indian woman is caught in a diabolical plot.

A painful mourning in acceptance of her condition, and recognition of her illusion of the analyst's omnipotence, allows a touch and contact to re-establish. The slow and tedious working through of a melancholic holding on makes way for the nascent beginnings of self again. This rebirth, premised on mourning the fantasy of medicine as the eradicator of herpes and the therapist as the eradicator of unwantedness, makes contact with reality conceivable. The analyst's eyes as witness to the patient's suffering work to refurbish a sense of self and are re-created as different from the policing and persecuting eyes of patriarchy. Our eyes, our seeing, and in the current context, screening, would perhaps always have the power to humiliate, to shun and look away when shamed. But the self, as able to take responsibility by appropriating and owning up to its needs and impulses (Sugarman, 2018), makes way for the patient to reclaim her sense of self and agency.

Notes

1 Herpes genitalis, caused by the herpes simplex virus type 1 or type 2, can manifest as primary or recurrent infection. Numerous studies have shown a significantly higher HSV-2 prevalence in women than in men. As a possible reason for this it has been suggested that men have asymptomatic genital HSV-2 infections more often than women resulting in higher transmission rates from men to women. Also genetic HSV-2 may remain asymptomatic in patients with HSV-1 immunity and vice versa. Till date there is no cure for the condition, however, immunotherapy (offered in some countries) can help with managing the condition (Sauerbrei, 2016).

2 For example, TB enhances sexual desire, while cancer is the disease of the sexually repressed. Additionally, the part of the body attacked in the scope of the illness, became the source of embarrassment and shame. TB, or cardiac illness, was not associated with shame and insult as much was cancer, for it attacked parts of the body (rectal, intestinal, ovarian) that induce shame and even repugnance.

3 Given that genital herpes can be caused by both variants of HSV, the mode of transmission is not contingent only on sexual intercourse. It can transmit by other modes; fellatio or cunnilingus (personal communication, Dr G. A. Mohan, MD Dermatology, Dr I. Mehraj, MD Dermatology).

4 The ego-ideal of Sita (her name meaning furrow, a universal symbol for the feminine genitalia) is a symbol of purity and devotion to one man – her husband. Her ideal plays an unconscious role as a defence against anxieties aroused by sexual impulses in the Indian woman's psyche (Kakar, 2012).

5 Intergenerationally transmitted eyes of Dharma make it acceptable for women to be sexual objects to a man but not sexual subjects (Narayanan, 2014).

Between contact and contagion 91

6 Patient details have been modified to protect confidentiality and maintain anonymity.
7 Herpes can remain largely asymptomatic and hence is not easily diagnosed (Staff, 2020).
8 The screen was placed diagonally behind the patient to re-create the therapy setting. We struggled with voice modulation in order to hear each other, finding the good enough (in her words, 'right position') distance that also made it possible for me to see her. The distance that humiliates also keeps from the bitter-sweet experience of intimacy.

References

Alizade, A. M. (1999). *Feminine sensuality*. H. Karnac (Books) Ltd.
Balsam, R. (2008). Sexuality and shame. *Journal of American Psychoanalytic Association*, 723–739.
Benjamin, J., & Atlas, G. (2015). The 'too muchness' of excitement: Sexuality in light of excess, attachment and affect regulation. *The International Journal of Psychoanalysis*, 96(1), 39–63.
Dimen, M. (2003). *Sexuality, intimacy, power*. The Analytic Press/Taylor & Francis Group.
Eigen, M. (2016). Shame. In M. Eigen (Ed.), *Image, sense, infinities, and everyday life* (pp. 61–86). Karnac Books.
Faimberg, H. (2005). *The telescoping of generations*. Routledge.
Haq, S. (2018). Sita through the time warp: On the ticklish relationship between renunciation and moral narcissism in the lives of young Indian women. In M. Kumar, A. Dhar, & A. Mishra (Eds.), *Psychoanalysis from the Indian terroir* (pp. 67–84). Lexington Books.
Haq, S. (2021). *In search of return mourning the disappearances in Kashmir*. Lexington Books.
Hartling, L. M., Rosen, W. B., Walker, M., & Jordan, J. V. (2004). Shame and humiliation: From isolation to relational transformation. In J. V. Jordan, M. Walker, & L. M. Hartling (Eds.), *The complexity of connection: Writings from the Stone Center's Jean Baker Miller Training Institute* (pp. 103–128). Guilford Press.
Herman, J. (2015). *Trauma and recovery*. Basic Books.
Kafka, F. (1981). *The metamorphosis* (S. Corngold, Trans.). Bantam Books.
Kakar, S. (1990). *Intimate relations*. Penguin Books.
Kakar, S. (2003). *Culture and psyche* (pp. 72–100). Oxford India Paperbacks.
Kakar, S. (2012). *The inner world*. Oxford India Perennials.
Kakar, S., & Kakar, K. (2007). *The Indians*. Penguin Random House India.
Mollon, P. (2005). The inherent shame of sexuality. *British Journal of Psychotherapy*, 22(2), 167–177.
Narayanan, A. (2014). Ambivalent subjects: Psychoanalysis, women's sexuality in India and the writings of Sudhir Kakar. *Psychodynamic Practice: Individual, Groups and Organisations*, 20(3), 213–227.
Pollock, G. (2006). Three essays on trauma and shame: Feminist perspectives on visual poetics. *Asian Journal of Women's Studies*, 12(4), 7–31.
Sauerbrei, A. (2016, October 18). ncbi.nlm.nih.gov/pmc/articles/PMC5177552/
Sontag, S. (1991). *Illness as metaphor and aids and its metaphors*. Doubleday.
Staff, M. C. (2020, October 13). www.mayoclinic.org/diseases-conditions/genital-herpes/symptoms-causes/syc-20356161

Steiner, J. (2011). *Seeing and being seen: Emerging from a psychic retreat*. Routledge.

Sugarman, A. (2018). The importance of promoting a sense of self-agency in child psychoanalysis. *The Psychoanalytic Study of the Child*, 71(1), 108–122.

Vanita, R. (2005). *Gandhi's tiger and Sita's smile; essays on gender, sexuality and culture*. Yoda Press.

8 Psychosocial reflections on destructiveness in the youth

Ashis Roy

The coronavirus has dictated life in a way that individuals and communities have not faced before. Social distancing, staying away from the workplace and keeping a distance from elders are actions and responses that are antithetical to the way individuals and social relations are structured in Indian society, which is overtly familial and relational in nature.

Such measures were taken for the first time, producing a difficult set of preoccupations that activated fears and beliefs within individuals which were often kept at bay in our modern-day existence. Under ordinary circumstances, these preoccupations are externally directed to threats and events 'outside' us rather than within us. Technology has played a vital role in helping people stay connected. However, it has also created a paradox between a self that could feel omnipotent and an emotional self that had to deal with many disturbing feelings and emotions. Even though individuals were being productive, they were also dealing with breakdowns within themselves which didn't find a space for expression and care in their functional lives. Many traumas that they encountered did not have a precedent, which could have enabled individuals to respond to them better.

This pandemic forced one to turn within one's body and mind (sanitizing one's dirt and craziness) and that created a claustrophobic helplessness and anxiety. The threat of getting infected, being the carrier of the virus or producing contagion through one's existence made this pandemic emotionally threatening. The panic created by the virus got translated within families: 'my closeness to my parents could cause them harm'.

As the pandemic unfolds and we look back, we find that it has left an indelible mark on the lives of many through chronic deaths, fatalities, families being wiped out and life being in constant danger for those who survived the virus.[1] Death penetrated every part of the social milieu and every interpersonal communication. There was no conversation in which death was not a participant. Unlike other tragedies like wars, tsunamis and riots, this one is peculiar in the mark that it will leave on people and on the state. The number of deaths, the suddenness with which it could completely ravage the self and the surroundings, would require a newer way of thinking about mourning, and loss, within the psyche.

DOI: 10.4324/9781003255895-9

Working within the context of the university I was able to see, at close quarters, such a crisis unfold where the functional educational self had to perform alongside emotional crises and life-changing circumstances. As online education kicked in, students had to perform their academic tasks as per schedule with some leeway provided by the university. Through various measures such as a helpline and communications through an online community, the mental health clinic in the university catered to students within the campus and members of the student community outside as they grappled with mental health issues that gradually became more acute. This was a new dialectic between the omnipotence that technology provided and the way it attempted to hide the crises at hand. The patients who had to shift to the online mode found it difficult to become subjects in the new virtual setting. It was assumed that each student and patient would be prepared to transfer themselves to the new medium and would be able to function equally well in the virtual space. Thus, just as the space of the physical clinic was replaced by the online clinic, where the setting was completely different and the change in the setting was an impingement (Ornston, 1978–1979) to the client, for a student to work in a context that was online without the physical presence of the teacher was also a task. It was taken for granted that the process of finding words, gathering one's thoughts and trusting one's mind had already taken place within the student as the student was asked to adapt to online teaching. Many students became quiet and their silence turned into withdrawal. Similarly, many patients found it hard to become subjects in this new space where they could not sense the somatic presence of their therapist. Psychoanalysis has been criticized for its denial of the body, and the present context made this denial more severe. However, technology also became a safe space, not contaminated by the virus but allowed human beings to interact and engage in these turbulent times. This complex relationship between technology and the psyche needs more attention and exploration. Technology challenges the *guru-shishya* relationship, which has been foundational in our civilization. The *shishya* (disciple) is now not so close to the environment, and the aura of the guru and the personal connection with the guru undergoes a change in this new environment.

The presence of *Ehsaas*[2] and its mental health resources allowed students to retain a safe caring relationship with the broken and fragmented parts in them. Particularly the space to be away from one's parents, which the adolescent desperately seeks, had disappeared. There was an absence of interaction with peers and teachers in ways that students were used to earlier. Additionally, this time saw an increase in interpersonal conflicts and violence at home.

One of my patients, Anubhav, a student suffering from diabetes, was undergoing an acute crisis. A political activist, his crisis included suicidal thoughts, an inability to concentrate and immense feelings of despair and helplessness. After a near-lethal suicide attempt, he approached the helpline. Listening to Anubhav, the sound of his voice told me that I was listening to a deeply fragmented soul. His thoughts were disconnected, often slipping away from each other and he sounded like he was constantly drowning into an abyss from where he needed rescuing. During this time, he had broken up with his girlfriend and a void had been created in his life. Academically he was struggling to finish his assignments.

Intense anger at his parents also made him feel alone and alienated. His parents didn't know what was happening within him. I have observed in several cases that when there is an emotional distance between a young person's internal state and his family's view of him, then the psychological distress gets intensified. States of breakdown need an active empathic imagination from within the family or else they become worse. Brief conversations with Anubhav's father helped me see him as a caring figure who wanted to do the best for his son. Symptoms are a language that gives expression to the self and often families don't have a way to understand the symptoms and emotions (Phillips, 1997). Due to the absence of a shared language to explain his inner world in his familial context, many experiences within Anubhav couldn't be expressed, for they didn't have a language. In my reveries, Anubhav experienced himself as Gregor Samsa from Kafka's short story 'Metamorphosis' (Kafka, 1915/2013), who was turning into something that no one could imagine. Metamorphosis evokes and captures the state of abjection (Kristeva, 2017) and sub-humanness in the human condition.

In Anubhav's experience, his parent's gestures of care towards him were humiliating. Often, he didn't have answers to their questions and he felt guilty that he was letting them down by not performing well academically. Much of the therapeutic work involved helping him face this internal pull of death, which evoked shame in him as he was ashamed of this part of himself that was in complete contradiction to his politically empowered self. The politically agentic self fought against state and institutional oppression, but within Anubhav also there was an oppressive environment that he struggled against.

The telephonic therapeutic alliance became a space where layers of shame could be witnessed and this enabled him to experience his vulnerability. Anubhav would often feel deeply persecuted and threatened when he was most helpless.

One day, as I was listening to him, I had a fantasy about my adorable dog, imagining her being bound in chains. Drawing from this, I said to him that 'at home you feel like a dog who is tied in chains'. I was scared while saying this as it could come across as being cruel and insensitive. Anubhav said, yes that's how I feel. It reassured me that we had enough faith that this shameful and threatened part of him could find an expression.

In acute psychic distress with his own mind pulling him down, Anubhav could not find inner structures that could make him feel stable. Green's (1999) description that the 'psyche can negate itself' describes similar mental states, which are governed by the work of the negative and inner destructiveness.

Affective deluge (Maltsberger, 1991) was predominant in his mind, and in those moments the family and the university became figures where his sense of mistrust could be lodged. In the absence of internal stable structures, other figures outside had to hold his persecutory projections. The fear of his own mind crumbling, disintegrating, was often too great, and seeing the university as an external source of fear was easier. Anubhav, however, always had the capacity to see both these layers even if at times he focused excessively on how the university, and perhaps in his experience the 'universe', had wronged him. For his agony to feel real and for him to feel less threatening to himself, someone on the outside had to be the one who had wronged him. This process of splitting (Feldman, 1992) was necessary for him to negotiate the difficult states within.

In his experience, because he didn't experience his mind as having distinct boundaries, others could torture him. Underlying this were, perhaps, deeper sadomasochistic fears of torture and humiliation.

The multiple layers of oppression that he experienced involved the experience of his inner state, the oppression of his parents, whose care felt like policing and humiliation, and the oppression of the university, which felt like the space that was making him anxious and depressed. Since the clinical work with Anubhav was not conventionally psychoanalytic, the possibility of exploring the intrapsychic and infantile origins of his trauma was limited. Often the university became the object that would be responsible for his inner oppression and turmoil. In the absence of a history of internal trauma and a sense of why he was suffering so much, the university had to become the structure that had failed him, in the absence of the inner structure/parent that had actually failed him. This sense of the university having failed him was conveyed through his experience of feeling scared that his teachers would not support him, whereas, on the contrary, his teachers thought of him as being bright and curious. Unfortunately, there was an absence of a positive internal object relationship in his internal world.

In the same period, the suicide of the famous Bollywood actor Sushant Singh Rajput was an awakening for him, as it was for many other patients. It reduced his shame around suicidal preoccupations. Suicidal attempts and thoughts were often his way of getting rid of intolerable states of mind (Eigen, 2019). In these phases, he would become more rageful and push everyone away. For Anubhav, therapy had to be a space that attended to this chaos and fragmentation within him where he would keep on collapsing. In his internal world, he was on a staircase where the stairs would keep disappearing. In my countertransference, I would experience him as a confused child dealing with contradictory mental states, needing attention and care, and my need to rescue him from the claustrophobic space that he experienced within. The child within him was also trying to negotiate the identity of an adult political activist, through which he derived an experience of an expansion of himself and his capacities.

The absence of the university as a space where he could channelize his aggression into creative political work would also aggravate his aggression. As this situation became grave, he felt more threatened that he would be unable to complete his educational degree and that the university would not support him. Thus, he would often experience life from the paranoid-schizoid position (Klein, 1946), which would create prolonged inertia. Our therapeutic relationship helped him see that he felt deeply unloved, scared of parts of his mind and couldn't trust a stable internal self. His mental contents found a holding space in therapy. I became a safe object through which he could see parts of himself with a lesser sense of persecution.

Although Anubhav had these issues that he was battling with, his struggle also indicated a larger fear that any student could feel about his vulnerabilities and states of breakdown being misunderstood within an academic setting where intellect is given precedence over other life circumstances and internal states of breakdown.

As a psychoanalytic thinker, I tried to think about which perspectives within psychoanalysis were more prudent for understanding the crisis, and I found that Klein's emphasis on destructiveness was useful as it reached into that core of the psyche that was feeling attacked both from within and without. As individuals had been turned into figures who could cause death to their loved ones, the presence of the self that cares had been withdrawn and it had been overtaken by a self that could damage the other person. Underlying people's need to be cautious there was also an internal claustrophobic anxiety of not knowing in which direction to move as the wish to care and the realization that one's presence could be damaging were both deeply intertwined.

Additionally, in an acute crisis, the patients in the clinic could feel that there was no container-contained (Bion, 1993) relationship that could introject their raw fears and dreads and give them back to them in a less harmful form. This experience was more prominent in patients whose need for survival was high, and psyche was already threatened.

The pandemic and online functionality created a split self which presumed that every individual could function efficiently in spite of experiencing breakdowns. An ignorance of mental health issues and a tendency to see them as anomalies can lead to a false sense that each individual is born with the capacity to deal with the possibility of death to others and to oneself. Unless the existence of these real fears of death and what they do to you is seen and provisions of care are created, many students and patients may suffer as they will be unable to feel integrated within themselves.

Notes

1 Survivor's guilt (Caruth & Lifton, 1991) is a phenomenon that needs to be studied in this context.
2 Low fee Psychoanalytic Psychotherapy Clinic at Ambedkar University Delhi.

References

Bion, W. R. (1993). *Attention interpretation*. Maresfield Library.

Caruth, C., & Lifton, R. (1991). Interview with Robert Jay Lifton. *American Imago*, 48(1), 153–175. Retrieved July 31, 2021, from www.jstor.org/stable/26304036

Eigen, M. (2019). *Toxic nourishment*. Routledge.

Feldman, M. (1992). Splitting and projective identification. In R. Anderson (Ed.), *Clinical lectures on Klein and Bion*. Tavistock/Routledge.

Green, A. (1999). *The work of the negative*. Free Association Books.

Kafka, F. (2013). *The metamorphosis* (S. Corngold, Trans.). Modern Library. (Original work published 1915)

Klein, M. (1946). Notes on some schizoid mechanisms. *The International Journal of Psychoanalysis*, 27, 99–110.

Kristeva, J. (2017). *Powers of horror: An essay on abjection*. Nota.

Maltsberger, J. T. (1991). The prevention of suicide in adults. In A. A. Leenaars (Ed.), *Life span perspectives of suicide: Time-lines in the suicide process* (pp. 295–307). Plenum Press.

Ornston, D. (1978–1979). Projective identification and maternal impingement. *International Journal of Psychoanalysis*, 7, 508–532.

Phillips, A. (1997). *Terrors and experts*. Harvard University Press.

9 The paradox of the COVID-19 event in Iran

At least we are not alone

Gohar Homayounpour

In the current global pandemic, Iran inhabits a unique position. Iran was one of the first countries to experience the outbreak (Jones & Wintour, 2020), while simultaneously having been the target of an ongoing economic blockade that has lasted for decades.

There has been a clear politicization of the COVID-19 pandemic, both from the Iranian government and by those outside of Iran who have used the current health crisis as yet another opportunity to politicize everything under the sun. So, in the middle of a pandemic, we are thrown into old, familiar and clichéd political games, once again completely oblivious of the Iranian people in general and, as always, the most forgotten classes of society in particular, who continue to be disregarded, left feeling alone and completely isolated.

When it comes to Iran, subject to continuous and long-lasting global and economic isolation, a clear split has been going on for decades, one which has had disastrous consequences for the people who live there. Change will only be possible if we start to work through this split, moving beyond consistent and comfortable binaries, beyond any axis of good or evil.[1] Possibly this tendency towards consistent and comfortable binaries is not specific to Iran, nor to the COVID-19 situation. Possibly it is, to some extent, the spirit of our times: this kind of concreteness reminiscent of our primary narcissism can be located right across our contemporary discourse of the politically correct: a part and parcel of the social liberal discourse. We search for consistencies and coherencies, often within a clichéd and concrete discourse of our times, forgetting that this search for consistency is merely achievable via the defensive function of splitting which inevitably leads to Bion's 'Attacks on Linking': 'the destructive attacks which the patient makes on anything which is felt to have the function of linking one object with another' (Bion, 1959). So not on the object but on linking.

I have had the privilege of hearing such a very diverse group of people's stories on my couch, which since the onset of the pandemic has been mostly online. It is my tendency for most of my psychoanalytic patients to use no video but only voice as our preferred mode during this particular time. There are certainly exceptions to this mode within my work, as always, considering the specific needs of each patient. What one can hear all over

DOI: 10.4324/9781003255895-10

our data are the universal concerns of COVID-19. Let's *listen* to some of these stories, not to psychoanalyse the various levels of each patient's psychic dynamics but, for the purpose of this chapter, to emphasize a specific point. It goes without saying that within the sessions one hears the patient's discourse according to her intrapsychic conflicts and unconscious fantasies, yet we must acknowledge the reality of the pandemic.

All over the data what is brought to the surface as a result of the current situation is: am I less or more alone? How connected or un-connected am I to others? In short reflections upon intimacies, these seem to be highlighted within the current reality.

Mrs A, who lives in the United States and has weekly sessions on the phone, expresses her delight; for now, all my other patients are also forced to use the phone. 'Now no one can come and lie on your couch', she says; as a result, she feels less isolated and alone.

Mrs M, whose birth was followed immediately by her father becoming severely ill with a highly infectious disease, is delighted at the sight of collective masking and social distancing laws, deep fears of contamination, of death, of fallen bodies. Suddenly the outside reality has perfectly matched her internal world, and the result is a deep sense of calm, connection to others and to the world. For the first time in her life, she feels as if she belongs, that she is not alone.

Mr E, who owns a cupcake store, was terrified of going bankrupt. 'Who would have the heart to buy such a non-essential item? Who would have the courage to risk contamination for an insignificant cupcake?' About eight months into the pandemic, he tells me:

> My estimation of how many cupcakes would sell was completely off. People kept buying them, even more than before, life goes on sweetly for some people. As for me, the bitter truth is that I lost eight kilos due to anxiety and fear of being contaminated, I am so sick, I feel so alone in my psychopathology. My state of psychic functioning is like the German joke that goes 'Why are the World Health Organization's rules dictating that we reduce the social distancing parameters we were already habitually practising?' Maybe I would feel less alone in Germany, I wonder if they continue to buy cupcakes there?

Mrs T, a hypochondriacal patient with various obsessive symptoms, tells me in her session: 'Now everybody's hands are like mine: I used to wash my hands so many times a day that they felt and looked like crocodile skin, but now we all have the same dry, disgusting-looking hands.'

I can hear all the psychoanalytic interpretations of my colleagues; however, I would like to emphasize, for the purposes of this chapter, the questions around feeling less/more alone as a repetitive common theme across what I assume many of us all over the world are hearing from patients, with a particularly heightened plot and twist in Iran due to its unique geopolitical situation and decades of isolation from the rest of the world.

Back to Mrs T: when the world became an emergency room, her usual state of psychic emergency became in sync with the world and all her usual anxieties left her. She kept saying: 'I was prepared. . . . I was well trained. . . . I am a capable human being, not a crazy one. . . . [N]ow all of the WHO's guidelines are what I was called crazy for all my life, my symptoms have become guidelines for others.'

Mr C says:

> I am so happy about the lockdown; I have always felt like I am 'missing out' on something; now everybody else is missing out with me; we are all missing out, which means I am not missing out, for you are only missing out if someone is not missing out; if everybody is missing out, then no one is. I feel great.

COVID-19 paradoxically took Mr C out of an internal sense of isolation. In a sense it seems to me that this is a shared sentiment of many Iranians these days. They felt fairly treated by COVID. I kept hearing from patients: 'Our children are less affected, just like everyone else, our elderly are more affected just like everywhere else in the world.' They felt treated justly by COVID. COVID did not name them as Iranian targets. The only difference, maybe the sole difference that remains in the imaginary, illusory taking away of all difference, is the difference between social classes, and yet that was visibly shown worldwide. COVID clearly hit the poor harder all over the world, from not having access to proper heath care to being more exposed to diabetes due to a less expensive, unhealthy diet, and forced to live with many people in small accommodations, and so on.

I believe the above examples could be a sample of what the pandemic could trigger according to the patient's unconscious fantasies, and, I assume, not so different from some of the associations analysts are hearing worldwide, with an emphasis on questions around intimacies.

Putting psychoanalysis to work, wishing/begging for a reciprocal contamination in this particular geography, I have been told by many patients since the beginning of the pandemic, time after time: 'At least now we are not alone.' Via the pandemic, Iranians are feeling a kinship, a linking, a sense of connection to the outside world. A kind of window out of their felt isolation. My patients keep saying: 'The whole world has the same enemy now, dealing with everyday, very similar struggles.' One patient said to me the other day:

> It is so comforting to see images of the entire world; suddenly the images are not so different to the reality of my everyday life in Iran. Everyone felt so distant before, now we are all together in this fight against the pandemic, it is as if borders have been taken away in sickness.

Or as another patient humorously elaborated on his joy of finding out the Iranian and American passports have become equally useless: 'Now, with either passport, you can't go anywhere.' He continued, saying that now everyone would comprehend what it is like to have a passport that you cannot travel easily with, what it feels like to be treated as if you already have a disease. Iranians were treated in such a way before the pandemic. 'At least we are all treated this way now.' Another patient said: 'It's so nice to see all governments failing all over the world, it is not just ours.'

A patient who has been experiencing extreme economic hardship as a result of the sanctions is finding a great deal of comfort in any news about the worldwide economic crisis. He keeps saying: 'At least I am not alone, at least Iran is not alone now, at least Iranians are not the only ones suffering anymore.'

A young girl associated, after she was infected with and recovered from COVID-19:

> You know, Doctor, throughout my illness I was feeling a sense of belonging to a community of people worldwide, I was part of a statistic that connected me to all those people of every nation, every colour, race and religion. I am so disgusted with international politics; why do we have to isolate a nation to such an extent that they would welcome a lethal virus as a way of belonging? Something is just not right about all of this. But as a COVID-19 patient, I felt a togetherness that I have not felt in a long time.

This link that has been possible to the outside world; this lineage through this virus has been very curative regarding the isolation Iranians have felt with regard to the world – this virus has become sort of a possibility of kinship, the linking that many all over the world feel deprived of by the virus and by the confinement. It has been greatly compensated for many people in Iran via 'At least we are not alone anymore', and this has lifted everyone's spirits to some extent, for we are not born to be alone, for we are desperately in search of connection, linking, linkage, even when our psychic sanctions make that very linkage the most terrifying encounter in the world.

We have to work through this terrorism of sanctions internally and externally, condemning it, no matter what the arguments in favour of it might be. Not in the name of sameness but that of difference. For sanctions will isolate, and we need to find our way to the outside world to develop a mind and to exist, without any illusionary wishes of universalization nor localization, but in the name of an encounter 'sans frontiers', a non-humanitarian hospitality towards ourselves and the other. Thus when a patient says, 'the current situation reminds me of a quote by Gore Vidal, "Every time a friend of mine succeeds something in me dies"', that is how many Iranians are feeling, that we have had to deal with a kind of COVID-19 for decades now (Cooke, 2015). Welcome to our world, for the quotation attributed to Vidal is not just about envy but, more primarily, a libidinal wish for kinship and lineage. Now we can be together.

I am by no means indicating that many of the losses, isolation, mourning, economic concerns were not part of the Iranian COVID-19 experience. These are certainly there, I am just trying to point that all over my patients' associations, there was also a paradoxical response of feeling connected to the outside world, feeling less lonely via the virus, which I think it is significant to elaborate both psychically and politically.

The pandemic is a disastrous event. I don't even join the optimism of those who assert this will help us to clean up the planet: humanity's memory is not its strongest suit; we will forget. But my patient will carry the pain of losing her mother without saying goodbye, a pregnant mother who lost her young husband to COVID-19 will remember her husband being robbed of meeting his first child, and millions of people will mourn deep losses, for, as Freud says about the loss of Sophie (his favourite daughter, whom he lost to the Spanish flu), '[t]his is not a way to die' (Rose, 2020).

This too shall pass. This is not the first pandemic nor will it be the last, and we will really only be able to say meaningful things after the storm has passed, and when our thinking thoughts have been to some extent restored. In the meanwhile, we deal with the deep fear/wish of connecting, wondering, dazed, why things have to get to such a dire state of isolation and fear for a nation that the arrival of a pandemic would be welcomed: a welcomed visitor for its citizens, who keep repeating on my couch here in Tehran 2020–2021, the years of the COVID-19 pandemic, that the virus spares no one, and in it, within it, we are reminded of our common human heritage, of our common fragility. This communal reminder and joint injury to our narcissism become a welcome messenger, a way of re-finding, in the final analysis, that we are all linked, in sickness and in health.

Note

1 A reference to President Bush's 2002 speech which named Iran along with Iraq and North Korea the 'axis of evil' (Bush, 2002).

References

Bion, W. R. (1959). Attacks on linking. *International Journal of Psychoanalysis, 40,* 308–316.

Bush, G. W. (2002, January 29). Text of President Bush's 2002 State of the Union Address. *The Washington Post.* Retrieved September 29, 2021, from www.washingtonpost.com/wp-srv/onpolitics/transcripts/sou012902.htm

Cooke, R. (2015). Every time a friend succeeds something inside me dies: The life of Gore Vidal by Jay Parini review – prurient and patronising. *The Guardian.* Retrieved December 16, 2020, from www.theguardian.com/books/2015/aug/23/every-time-a-friend-succeeds-something-inside-me-dies-the-life-of-gore-vidal-by-jay-parini-review

Jones, S., & Wintour, P. (2020, March 6). 'Coronavirus cases pass 100,000 globally as Iran threatens force to restrict travel.' *The Guardian.* www.theguardian.com/world/2020/mar/06/chinese-schools-reopen-as-coronavirus-cases-in-europe-continue-to-rise

Rose, J. (2020). To die one's own death. *London Review of Books, 42*(22).

10 What does therapy look like in times of lockdown? A view from Paris

Anne Gagnant de Weck and Benjamin Lévy

Introduction

In France, strict health rules and lockdown measures due to the health crisis were decreed in a rather harsh and sudden way in the middle of March 2020. Whereas Italy, a neighbouring country, had progressively been confined from 21 February, the French could not imagine that they would find themselves in such a situation. When, on Thursday 12 March, President Emmanuel Macron announced that nurseries, schools and universities would be closed, the whole country was astonished. Over the next three days, the French prepared for lockdown: they organized remote work, they cleaned out the food stores, and those who had a country house left their flat in the city. On Monday 16 March, in a ceremonial speech, Emmanuel Macron declared lockdown from the next day at noon. People had to stay within one kilometre of their homes and could not meet others, even in private places, unless they had a valid reason to do so (such as going to work when the work was considered to be essential and important and working remotely was not possible, providing vital supplies or emergency help to the most vulnerable ones, providing medical consultations which could not be provided online). Like everyone else, psychoanalysts had to choose a place to confine themselves and to find new ways of working from home. The lockdown lasted from 17 March to 11 May.

To report on this unprecedented period, we have relied largely on 18 in-depth interviews with psychoanalysts (10 men and 8 women) carried out through Zoom by film directors Clovis Stocchetti and Pascal Laethier, the latter also a psychoanalyst (Laethier & Stocchetti, 2020).[1] These interviews show the contributors' reactions, the solutions they adopted and their observations on psychoanalysis during lockdown. We have also read several dozen papers published in major French journals of psychology, psychiatry or psychoanalysis, plus several dozen contributions to the blogs of some French psychoanalytical institutions which had created spaces for their members to express themselves. Finally, so as to make a comparison with the situation in other countries and determine whether there were any differences between therapists confronted with the lockdown in France and

DOI: 10.4324/9781003255895-11

outside France, we have consulted the websites of non-French analytical institutions and the publications of their members on their blogs or in specialized journals.[2]

An experimental period

Reactions of the analysts

Video testimonials and articles written by therapists on blogs attest to their great resourcefulness in finding answers and solutions when confronted with the impossibility of continuing face-to-face therapy. Some therapists, representing a small minority, initially refused to continue follow-ups with their patients through electronic devices. Some insisted that the presence of the body was vital to analytical practice, while some emphasized the importance of their workplace as the framework of the analytical ritual. It should be noted that some of these opponents to remote analysis have subsequently adopted teleworking, sometimes – they say – at the request of their patients. A second group is composed of those who, already accustomed to remote consulting, have simply systematized this practice. They did not see it as something really new. Between these two extremes, most therapists appear to have reluctantly resigned themselves to the use of remote analysis. During lockdown, they have sometimes discovered the benefits of such a practice, or at least got used to it. Among them, some preferred to use the phone only and not Skype or Zoom because of the fear of the fascination effect induced by the digital image.[3]

In this group of therapists – who have recently converted to remote analysis – resourcefulness seems to have been the greatest. Some called their patients, while others waited for their patients to call them. A few seconds before their appointment, some patients had to send a short message indicating that they were 'in the waiting room', after which the therapist would text to say that he or she was available for a call. Teleconsultations, Zoom, Facetime or Skype have sometimes been adapted to maintain a frame or even a semblance of rituality, for example, through the re-creation of a formal setting (with an armchair, books in the background and so on).

Being medical doctors, psychoanalysts who were also practising as psychiatrists could provide a certificate allowing for in-person therapy. A few non-psychiatric analysts also made the choice to continue receiving certain patients in a way that was not entirely legal. This choice was the subject of fierce controversy in discussion groups among colleagues, because of the health risk involved, the risk of patients arriving at the consulting room being checked by the police, and the risk of a fine. It has been defended by some as the patients' free choice to accept this solution, and as a way of preserving the distinctiveness of psychoanalysis from any standard medical practice.

The variable role of institutions

The resourcefulness shown by some French analysts may be partly linked to the fact that most of them evolve on the periphery of Lacanian institutions. They are no strangers to these, since they attend them for seminars and training activities, but neither are they integrated into a rigid hierarchy which distributes institutional ranks and functions. As a result, Lacanian institutions have rather limited control over analytical practices, including those of therapists who are involved with them. They may set up discussion groups, seminars or blogs where everyone can intervene, but it is not their policy to establish rigid standards that apply to everyone.

This contrasts sharply with psychoanalytic institutions affiliated to the IPA, which are a minority in France. In fact, the IPA has fully modified its official web-page so as to tackle the clinical challenge represented by the lockdown (International Psychoanalytical Association, *Practising psychoanalysis and psychotherapy during a time of crisis: coronavirus (COVID-19)*, n.d.). Members of the IPA were not only invited to contribute to blogs or offered spaces for collegial discussion but also received some advice for surviving the coronavirus-induced isolation, or they could watch an impressive number of webinars and read precise guidelines about remote sessions and their confidentiality (International Psychoanalytical Association, *Videos*, n.d.). The IPA, therefore, sought to regulate this practice, creating a new global standard for lockdown times.

As we have said, French-Lacanian institutions have adopted the opposite attitude. Although they switched their seminars to Zoom, some tended to deny that there was anything new to think about, because a minority of analysts had already been using remote therapy for a long time, even if only marginally until then. The IPA attitude of regulating the new system and setting up guidelines is, thus, in sharp contrast to the Lacanian position, being nearer 'Nothing moves and nothing stirs in the analytical realm, which keeps being itself whatever happens'.

Discussion groups and blogs

Independent of the reaction of institutions, the lockdown created a sudden need for new thoughts and renewed considerations about psychoanalysis. In the French-Lacanian context, these new thoughts have often been shared through 'cartels' now organized on Skype or Zoom. The importance of the 'cartel' for French- Lacanian psychoanalysis must here be underlined (see, for instance, Adam, 2003). It is a horizontal and flexible group with a small number of participants (usually around five) who gather about once a month in a half-informal context. In normal times, their members would often share a dinner followed by a discussion about a book, a text or a topic chosen in advance. Well adapted to Skype or Zoom meetings, this format of half-informal small-group discussions has proved to be very resilient in times of crisis.

All in all, a good number of small- to medium-sized non-IPA psycho-analytical institutions in Paris and other French towns have invented new virtual spaces and times dedicated to questions about the lockdown and analytical practice, be it through blogs or remote seminars.[4] In fact, at the local level, virtually every practitioner has had opportunities to discuss these topics and write articles whenever they felt the need to do so. These articles can be distributed into three categories: (1) psychoanalytical considerations about the global pandemic and the civilizational crisis it fostered, (2) some technical thoughts about analytical practice and its settings during the pandemic and (3) clinical studies about reactions to the lockdown and changes of psychic functioning in patients. This gave rise to a flowering of articles testifying to the vitality of analytical practice.

Changes in the setting

Overnight, therapists who had not anticipated the lockdown had to adapt and find viable alternatives to allow for follow-ups. After two or three days of uncertainty, most psychoanalysts phoned or wrote to their patients, either to explain to them how therapy would go on during lockdown or to ask them what they wanted to do in such an unusual situation and thus build a new setting together. Some therapists felt that *conditions had been reversed*: suddenly, psychoanalysts had to call their patients and ask them to stay on in therapy in spite of the lockdown (Laethier & Stocchetti, 2020; Lombardi, 2021; and more generally Levine & de Staal, 2021, in parts III and IV of the book). Some psychoanalysts felt uncomfortable doing this as it seemed as if they 'needed' their patients. Obviously, such a reversal is likely to have consequences on transference.

In some institutions, however, where patients are referred to therapists by schools or by social services and do not always come willingly on their own, this reversal in 'who appears to ask for therapy' had sometimes ben-eficial effects on therapeutic work. One female psychoanalyst working with children and teenagers in a medical centre explained that while usually the centre insists that the request must come from patients, even when this is obviously not the case, the remote therapy practised during lockdown some-how set the record straight: patients did not want to come, but the social services had asked them to do so. As a therapist, she took the responsibility of being the one who came to them, who called them, who cared for them, who wanted to keep in touch during this crisis. According to her, taking the responsibility for continuing the therapy dispelled the illusion of the patients coming by themselves – something no one truly believes – and established a healthier relationship with some patients, who were heartened and touched by her support during these difficult times.

Generally, therefore, therapists had to reinvent their practices in no time. These sudden rearrangements may have urged some patients to stop their therapy, but few therapists *faced* massive desertions. Most of them pointed out that at least 50 per cent of their patients stayed, while some said almost all of them stayed. For the patients who stayed, going from conventional therapy to remote therapy caused very tangible changes in the therapeutic setting. These changes, in turn, had consequences on the therapeutic work itself. We will now describe this new configuration.

Absence of bodies

First of all, with remote therapy, the co-presence of bodies in the same space disappears. Only the voice remains – and the image in the case of videoconferencing, but this image can by no means be compared with the real presence of bodies. Remote therapy is based on a wholly different type of presence as compared to face-to-face therapy, as has been shown by two examples of remote cures with children by de Mello (2021) and Durban (2021). Faced with this dramatic change, therapists had different reactions. A small number of them maintained that the voice is a full and in no way lessened presence and that remote therapy does not suffer from deficiencies and impairments when compared to conventional therapy. These therapists insist that the cure is not dependent on a fixed setting (the couch-chair system) and can be carried out in a wide variety of circumstances, as long as the transference is established and the psychoanalyst's desire supports the cure (see, for example, Lippi, 2020). One female psychoanalyst said: 'The setting is above all a psychic place, in which the transferential relationship is elaborated. And the psychoanalyst is the guarantor of this setting.' The setting is thus visualized as a psychic and not a physical place. Two psychoanalysts pointed out that Freud himself sometimes practised in very different circumstances from those that were subsequently established as the conventional setting, for example, during his cure with Ferenczi, which was largely carried out during walks. Freud's therapeutic discussion with the composer Gustav Mahler, which also took place during a walk, was also quoted in support of this viewpoint.

Conversely, other therapists, few in number as well, could not imagine practising remote therapy. For them, the cure was wholly dependent on a ritualized setting, without which there could be no real therapeutic work. The co-presence of bodies was not optional, it was a *sine qua non* condition for real psychoanalytical work, because, for talking to impose itself as the only linchpin of therapy, touch or sight must be *available* but *forbidden*. A male psychoanalyst summed up this idea, saying: 'One of the basic principles of our beautiful profession is the prohibition of touching. What happens to the prohibition of touching when you precisely cannot touch?' The shift from the forbidden to the impossible, resulting from the absence of the body, creates a fundamentally different relationship to fantasy and to the law and does not establish talking as the only *authorized* therapeutic means. The other drives must remain accessible in order to be prohibited. One female therapist also noticed that psychoanalysis is often blamed for neglecting the body, whereas the body must actually be present but its use must be regulated within the psychoanalytical setting.[5] As a result, the absence of the body changes the instinctual energy set in motion when talking, and jouissance does not circulate in the same way in transference. Therapists convinced of the necessary co-presence of bodies sometimes chose not to continue working with their patients during lockdown or to work in their consulting rooms in spite of the prohibition of leaving one's home, either because, as doctors, they were able to issue medical discharge certificates to their patients or because they just decided to break the law. Some of them sometimes agreed to have their patients on the phone, but they insisted that this was in no way psychoanalysis, but just a kind of support for patients in distress.

Most therapists, however, fell somewhere in between. While they noticed significant differences between remote and face-to-face therapy, and thought the latter preferable, they did not refuse to keep practising during lockdown, nor did they consider remote therapy to be devoid of qualities. Many therapists admitted that they were pleasantly surprised to be able to keep doing really good therapeutic work over the phone or by videoconference (for another interesting testimony see Roth, 2020). This is not to say that the absence of the bodies does not have significant effects on both the psychoanalyst and the patient. On the patient's side, the absence of the analyst's gaze seems to have had contradictory consequences. For some, not being under the gaze of the therapist had a liberating effect. It created a distance which enabled them to free themselves from a feeling of shame and to talk about things they had not yet dared to talk about. One psychoanalyst explains that she first heard about a patient's sexual abuse on the telephone. Not being seen enabled her to talk about it. For other patients, on the contrary, the absence of the analyst's gaze had an inhibiting effect. These patients needed a supportive gaze to be able to speak. The naked voice of the therapist, in its dry and disembodied state, cannot provide this imaginary support. Whether invasive or protective, the psychoanalyst's gaze plays a key role in therapy, and its absence changes what can or cannot be said.

On the psychoanalyst's side, the absence of the patient's body had various effects on their ways of listening. Several psychoanalysts said that they were more easily distracted during phone sessions. Without the support of physical presence, their minds tended to wander and follow their own thoughts, in a way that they did not overlap with the 'floating attention' during analytical listening. Some therapists implemented strategies to deal with their distraction. One psychoanalyst said that he began to write down what his patients said in order to compel himself to listen to them attentively. Others noticed that some positions were much more conducive to listening. Many said they walked a lot during the sessions, as the pace of walking allowed for floating attention. A few of them, on the contrary, preferred to be comfortably seated on their sofas during the sessions. One psychoanalyst said that she had listened to some of her patients lying down, in the position normally reserved for patients. In any case, many therapists seem to have appreciated the freedom of movement allowed by remote therapy. For instance, one female psychoanalyst remarked:

> I realized that I put a lot of energy into staying still. That is to say that during a session, it is sometimes hard for me to stay still. And here, I felt completely free to move around. . . . I realized that because I could move, I was not focused on the fact that I had to stay still. And so, I was a better listener.

If some therapists appreciated being away from their patients, some could also miss their physical presence. Distance therapy prevents non-verbal communication. The way of greeting the patient, of looking at him or her, of shaking his or her hand to say goodbye and so on, all these relational modalities disappear with remote therapy, and some therapists have felt deprived of a valuable means of communication.[6] A psychoanalyst says, for example, that after a particularly difficult session, she finds a way to discreetly say 'good luck' to the patient, without formulating it explicitly: she shakes hands more firmly than usual, putting her second hand over the patient's hand. These small tokens of empathy and support, which can be very important in transference, are no longer possible in remote therapy. In the absence of the body, talking becomes even more central, almost exclusive.

Finally, remote therapy has sometimes had the paradoxical effect of making one feel closer to the other's body. According to several therapists, this is especially true with phones. Having the other person's voice whispered in your ear brings about an intimacy that may be disturbing. Uncomfortable with this excessive intimacy, further accentuated by the fact that the patient's voice is heard from a private space, one psychoanalyst began using the loudspeaker to restore distance. Remote therapy can, therefore, bring about a greater porosity between the private and the public, and requires strategies to maintain the distance between the two.

Absence of a common place

In remote therapy, both therapists and patients have to deal with the disappearance of the consulting room as a neutral place, belonging to neither of them, where the encounter is made possible because social roles and identifications are put in brackets and the noise of the world is suspended. On the contrary, everyone joins remote therapy from a private space, usually from home. Even more, with image – but also, to a lesser extent, with sound alone – one goes into the other's home as much as the other comes into theirs. This leads to a distortion of spaces and has been felt to be intrusive by many psychoanalysts who, for this reason, felt more comfortable with the phone than with image-based media. Some therapists did not wish to be seen in their private space. Others were even more embarrassed to enter their patients' homes. On the patients' side, if many felt uncomfortable as well, some, especially among the young, enthusiastically embraced this blurring between private and public space. A male psychoanalyst working in a medical centre explains, for example, that a teenager was delighted to be able to take his camera and show him what was in his home (for similar examples, see de Mello, 2021, and Durban, 2021). This brought the therapist closer to him and helped strengthen their relationship. Another psychoanalyst, also working in one of these centres, was surprised to find that phone therapy worked very well with a complicated, hyperactive child who was constantly on the move and had difficulty talking in face-to-face therapy. It was as if the absence of the body enabled him to engage in the talking.

Among therapists, however, there was a shared sense of bringing down a necessary boundary for therapeutic work. Therapy is supposed to take place in a setting that is largely impervious to the external world, as if the patient and the therapist are suddenly cut off from their daily lives. Therapy therefore presupposes an operation of cutting oneself from one's life and moving to another forum, what psychoanalysts call the 'other scene', where transference is carried out. With remote therapy, the very possibility of an enclosed and sealed space seems to be jeopardized, for daily life has more opportunity to break into the therapy. This sometimes led to unusual situations, to say the least, such as this patient, mentioned by a psychoanalyst, who had a phone session while shopping in a supermarket, or this psychoanalyst who listened to his patients while walking in his neighbourhood and who, in the middle of a session, was arrested by the police for a check on his exit permit (a small piece of paper justifying the reason for leaving one's home, which all French people had to carry when leaving their places of confinement).

During lockdown, the absence of a common physical place has had, as its intrapsychic equivalent, the disappearance or at least the displacement of this 'other scene', that of the unconscious, where the free associations of the analysand can be elaborated. The absence of a neutral space where the encounter is made possible was echoed by a quasi-absence of free associations in the patients' discourse. A large proportion of therapists testified that their patients had a clear tendency to 'discuss' rather than freely associate, which barely allowed them to extricate themselves from the thread of current events and from a state of dazed astonishment.[7]

Even when the lockdown was over and analysts gradually resumed their activities in their office, certain restrictive health standards dictated by the government continued to apply. Was it necessary to cover the couch with a sheet, keep the mask on for the entire session, wash hands and disinfect furniture after each appointment? Implicit in these was the question of whether the practice is a private place, where intimate things are said, far from the public space and imposed norms, or whether it is a public place, where the rules that govern other public spaces and the concerns that go with them also apply.

The intrusion of reality in the cure

Sharing tough times together

Because of the health crisis, some patients and therapists had the strong impression that they were going through something serious together (see Levine & de Staal, 2021, especially parts I and III; and Kushwaha, 2020). During the sessions, external events brought out concerns for the health of the analyst, the patient and their loved ones, but it was rarely possible to analyse the unconscious reasons for such concerns. Under normal circumstances, they could have been the object, if not of interpretation, at least of a silent distancing on the part of the analyst. Such a silence in these circumstances could become intolerable. A demand for empathetic participation in collective suffering was presented to the therapist and refusing this empathy, far from being perceived as an ethical act allowing the preservation of an analytical framework separate from everyday concerns, was tantamount to a kind of betrayal of the patient. As a result, an unusual curiosity seems to have become the norm. Some questions may have emerged without being considered testimonies of the patient's fantasy activity, for example, when asking where the analyst was confined and with whom. To ask such questions would normally have been inappropriate, but suddenly seemed legitimate.

The situation could also cause particular resentment, for example, if a patient realized that his therapist had left the town where he normally practised. This was in keeping with the commonly held belief of the time that the richest (and most irresponsible) citizens were fleeing the unhealthy city to retreat to comfortable country homes, leaving the poorest to their fate. A whole set of questions that the analyst would normally have indicated as fantasy was thus projected onto the scene of reality without the patient always being able to detach himself from it.

All in all, the imposed distancing caused an attack on the analyst-patient link and rekindled resistance that was often masked by benevolent attitudes.

A casual conversation?

Because many of the concerns that belong outside the sessions suddenly found a place in them, many psychoanalysts noticed that remote sessions often transformed themselves into ordinary conversations. Patients and therapists would check in with each other with 'Hello, how are you?' Both the language used and the symmetry established between therapist and patient are far removed from the usual mode of interaction in therapy, and even more so in psychoanalytically oriented therapy. The psychoanalyst, as a private person, suddenly took on an importance that he is not supposed to have in normal times. Many therapists have accepted, to varying degrees, not to be just a role and a function but to take on their real personhood, so to speak.

The health crisis, being deeply unusual, overwhelmed certain sessions, which became wholly focused on current events, thus bringing the words exchanged between therapists and patients even closer to an ordinary conversation between friends in COVID time. Several therapists shared that they experienced much difficulty in driving some patients away from such invasive and disturbing news (see Schinaia, 2020). Likewise, several therapists said that they had difficulty hearing a signifier over the phone or by videoconference. They found it difficult to go beyond the explicit meaning of what was said and to hear something other than what was overtly being said through the patient's words (Laethier & Stocchetti, 2020; Blondel, 2020). Because of the extraordinary circumstances, they felt caught up in the meaning of the statements and bogged down in the common discourse. One male therapist said, for example, that he felt 'caught up, in spite of himself, in a concern for the other that puts him in an intentionally aimed practice'.

No room for meaningful silences

In addition to the more ordinary and more meaning-driven talking, it is the rhythm and pace of the session that varies greatly in remote therapy. Many psychoanalysts pointed out a different distribution of silence and talking. In particular, silences had neither the same place nor the same meaning over the phone or in videoconferencing. Using a technical means had, indeed, an important consequence: it was difficult, if not impossible, to make out the difference between an intentional silence – a sign of listening and attention on the therapist's side, of rhythm and meaning on the patient's side – and the silence that came from a technical problem. On the phone or by videoconference, when faced with silence, the natural reaction is to say 'Hello?' to make sure that the communication has not been cut off. For this reason, many therapists noticed that they were spontaneously led to use much more phatic expressions – little words with no other purpose than keeping communication going: hum, yes, I see, okay, alright and so on. In doing so, they simply meant that they were present and listening.

Similarly, due to the inevitable small time lags between the issuer and the recipient on the phone or by videoconference, some therapists said they had difficulty inserting an incision in the patient's talking, repeating a word, suggesting a small adjustment to this or that term, asking for clarification. The interlacing of the therapist's talk with the patient's is much more difficult in remote therapy. For this reason, these therapists tended either to keep silent, barely pronouncing small words to mark their presence, or to speak in a longer and more developed way. Many therapists noticed that they were much more talkative on the phone than in face-to-face sessions. The absence of physical presence seems to be compensated by a reinforced presence of the voice.

Money distanced

With the absence of bodies and the dematerialization of sessions, the question of payment also became important. Payment is an important moment in the session, which, far from being considered as a mere formality, is the subject of many reflections in psychoanalytical circles. Some therapists want their patients to pay in cash. If the payment has a tangible reality, patients will become aware of what they are spending to get better and they will not feel indebted to the therapist who helps them in this therapeutic process. Others accept cheques. Few, however, offer to accept payment by bank transfer. In any case, the payment is also about the patient's investment in the therapy and his or her relationship with the therapist. It must therefore be given a close look. During lockdown, most therapists chose to either ask the patient to make a wire transfer to them, sometimes hiding their address on the bank identity number they sent to their patients, or let their patients' debt accumulate, which they would settle when they went back to the office. In both cases, money seems to have become more distant, less tangible, not only dematerialized but sometimes long delayed. Because of distancing in payment, remote therapy is even more likely to appear like an ordinary conversation between friends.

Conclusion: Towards a more democratic setting?

The lockdown forced therapists to reinvent their practices in a matter of days, creating ideal conditions for multiple experiments that would not have been possible in normal times. Many therapists say that they have enjoyed breaking free from the classical setting and experimenting with other arrangements. The feeling of being caught unprepared and helpless, following the announcement of the lockdown, often gave way, after some time, to a feeling of freedom and great inventiveness. The huge number of testimonies published on blogs, in journals and books – or even in the form of films – testifies in itself to this great inventiveness and reflects this sudden feeling of creative freedom.

However, the novelty of the practices used by therapists during lockdown should not be exaggerated. This extraordinary period has brought to light some things that, until then, were done discreetly. It has revealed, as a basic trend, the softening of the classical psychoanalytical setting. Just a few years before the global pandemic, this trend had already been acutely described by Antonino Ferro, former president of the Italian psychoanalytic society (Ferro, 2017). This seems to be correlated with the much less vertical (authority) and much more horizontal (intersubjectivity) dimension of the patient-to-therapist relationship that has been established over the last 20 or 30 years. The development of intersubjectivist tendencies in Anglo-Saxon psychoanalysis is only one facet of this important movement, which can also be linked to the rise of a form of 'health democracy'. It induces fundamental changes in style and inspires trends as diverse as the critique of patriarchy, convergences between psychoanalysis and gender studies or interactions with postcolonial studies (see, for instance, Ayouch, 2018, and on an even more controversial note, Greedharry, 2008). In the wake of this, the aura of psychoanalysts – once seen as intellectuals as well as therapists – has been reduced. Patients seem to expect therapists to be more empathetic, democratic and less intellectual and paternal than before (Ferro, 2017; Ayouch, 2018; Greedharry, 2008). In other words, they expect more horizontal interactions with their analyst, something for which remote sessions are rather appropriate.

Notes

1 This self-funded documentary has been displayed online on Vimeo and discussed at several psychoanalytical video-meetings.
2 More details about these blogs and websites are given below. In June 2020, the *Journal of the American Psychoanalytic Association* released a special issue on Psychoanalysis and the Pandemic (vol. 68(3)).
3 There are dozens of documents on the topic tackled in this paragraph. It is discussed in Laethier and Stocchetti's film; some articles have also been written by French psychoanalysts and exchanged on blogs (see the following). Lastly, see Levine and de Staal (2021), Chherawala and Gill (2020) and Antonino Ferro (Ferro, 2021)
4 See the blogs of French associations Psychanalyse actuelle (2020) and FEDEPSY (2020). In the IPA sphere, a huge diversity of articles have also been written and a blog dedicated to the pandemics has been created: www.ipa.world/IPA/en/News/corona_papers.aspx
5 See also Levine and de Staal (2021), in particular the chapters by Chervet (2021) and Barros and Barros (2021).
6 Apart from Laethier and Stocchetti's film see, for instance, contributions by Aline Mizrahi and Isabelle Carré on Psychanalyse Actuelle's blog (2020).
7 This topic is discussed in Laethier and Stocchetti's film. For similar examples given by Chinese therapists and patients, see Zhao Ming's and Lijing's contributions on Psychanalyse Actuelle's blog (2020).

References

Adam, J. (2003). L'opération cartel. *Essaim*, 1(11), 165–170.

Ayouch, T. (2018). *Psychanalyse et hybridité: genre, colonialité, subjectivations.* Leuven University Press.

Barros, A. R., & Barros, E. R. (2021). Landscapes of mental life under Covid-19. In H. B. Levine & A. de Staal. (Eds.), *Psychoanalysis and Covidian life* (pp. 61–81). Phoenix Publishing House.

Blondel, P.-E. (2020). *Le cabinet vidé des corps.* https://fedepsy.org/wp-content/uploads/2020/04/EPHEMERIDE-2-Pierre-%C3%89douard-Blondel.pdf

Chervet, B. (2021). The shattering of a denial as food for thought. In H. B. Levine & A. de Staal (Eds.), *Psychoanalysis and Covidian life* (pp. 39–59). Phoenix Publishing House.

Chherawala, N., & Gill, S. (2020). Up-to-date review of psychotherapy via videoconference: Implications and recommendations for the RANZCP Psychotherapy Written Case during the COVID-19 pandemic. *Australasian Psychiatry*, 28(5), 517–520.

De Mello, P. C. (2021). Where does the psychoanalyst live? The online setting in the psychoanalysis of a three-year-old girl on the autistic spectrum. In H. B. Levine &

A. de Staal (Eds.), *Psychoanalysis and Covidian life* (pp. 219–241). Phoenix Publishing House.

Durban, J. (2021). Where does the Covid live? Osmotic/diffuse anxieties, isolation, and containment in times of the plague. In H. B. Levine & A. de Staal (Eds.), *Psychoanalysis and Covidian life* (pp. 243–259). Phoenix Publishing House.

Fédération Européenne de Psychanalyse et Ecole Psychanalytique de Strasbourg (FEDEPSY). (2020). https://fedepsy.org/2020/04/07/ephemeride-1-le-journal-du-confinement/

Ferro, A. (2017). *The new analyst's guide to the galaxy: Questions about contemporary psychoanalysis*. Routledge.

Ferro, A. (2021). Being online: What does it mean for psychoanalysis? In H. B. Levine & A. de Staal (Eds.), *Psychoanalysis and Covidian life* (pp. 99–105). Phoenix Publishing House.

Greedharry, M. (2008). *Postcolonial theory and psychoanalysis. From uneasy engagements to effective critique*. Palgrave Macmillan.

International Psychoanalytical Association. (n.d.-a). *Practising psychoanalysis and psychotherapy during a time of crisis: Coronavirus (COVID-19)*. www.ipa.world/IPA/en/News/coronavirus.aspx

International Psychoanalytical Association. (n.d.-b). *Videos*. www.ipa.world/IPA/en/News/corona_videos.aspx

Kushwaha, A. (2020). *W(a/o)ndering with the virus*. https://thepsychotherapistcollective.in/blog/waondering-with-the-virus/

Laethier, P., & Stocchetti, C. (Directors). (2020). *Psychanalyse et psychanalystes au temps du confinement*. Self-Financed.

Levine, H. B., & de Staal, A. (Eds.). (2021). *Psychoanalysis and Covidian life*. Phoenix Publishing House.

Lippi, S. (2020). *Télé-psychanalyse: le transfert au temps du Corona*. https://aoc.media/opinion/2020/06/02/tele-psychanalyse-le-transfert-au-temps-du-corona/

Lombardi, R. (2021). Body and souls in remote analysis: Anguished countertransference, pandemic panic and space-time limits. In H. B. Levine & A. de Staal (Eds.), *Psychoanalysis and Covidian life* (pp. 143–160). Phoenix Publishing House.

Psychanalyse actuelle. (2020). www.psychanalyseactuelle.com/le-blog/all%C3%B4-all%C3%B4-vous-mentendez

Roth, M. (2020). *Transference in the time of corona*. www.ipa.world/IPA/en/News/corona_papers.aspx

Schinaia, C. (2020). *Psychoanalysis in the age of coronavirus*. www.ipa.world/IPA/en/News/corona_papers.aspx

11 The waves of loss

Surabhika Maheshwari

The last couple of years have seen the world go through unimaginable flux – COVID-19 and its lockdowns brought about a complete change in life, relationships, routines, home, and work as we once knew it. Reliable ways of negotiating our realities and the world came to a halt and we have been locked up with the dread of the illness looming large. The virus – a highly infectious one – could and was infecting everybody. It wouldn't be an exaggeration to say that the impact of the coronavirus is beyond getting infected and we have no statistics to address the effect on all those who have suffered during the pandemic even without really 'being infected by the virus'. On 31 December 2019 WHO was informed of cases of pneumonia of unknown cause in Wuhan City, China. A novel coronavirus was identified as the cause by Chinese authorities on 7 January 2020 and was temporarily named '2019-nCoV'. On 30 January 2020 Dr Tedros Adhanom Ghebreyesus, WHO director-general, declared the novel coronavirus outbreak a public health emergency of international concern, WHO's highest level of alarm. At that time there were 98 cases in 18 countries outside China and no deaths. On 11 March 2020, the rapid increase in the number of cases outside China led the WHO director-general to announce that the outbreak could be characterized as a pandemic. By then more than 1,18,000 cases had been reported in 114 countries, and 4291 deaths had been recorded (WHO, 2020). The spread was rapid and the illness began to take mammoth proportions. A world pulsating with scientific progress and striding ahead with ever-new inventions, shrinking with rapid and complete connectivity was held hostage to a virus that was threatening to break all order. And it did. Without warning or preparation, in less than 30 days, it became a deadly scare travelling rapidly around the globe. With the spread of the virus came immediate efforts to contain it and lockdowns were announced. Well over 100 countries worldwide instituted either a full or partial lockdown by the end of March 2020, affecting billions of people. When the virus first appeared, several countries brought in initial restrictions on flights from China, or required visitors from at-risk areas to be quarantined on arrival. By the end of March, air traffic from some of the world's biggest airports had dropped to a fraction of what it had been at the same time the year before,

DOI: 10.4324/9781003255895-12

or even what it had been at the start of the month. Travel within major cities across the globe ground to a halt as restrictions on movement and social contact came into force (BBC, 2020). The precipitous beginning and the unprecedented outbreak led each one of us to be drawn into the pandemic in myriad ways – getting infected, seeing loved ones infected, living through lockdowns, living with changing protocols, adjusting to new guidelines, not seeing loved ones, not meeting people we had met regularly earlier, the world moving further away, losing jobs, financial stress, being bombarded with news of loss and grief, witnessing the pandemic move closer and bigger, having to move cities to accommodate work and caregiving.

The inescapability of loss

In the context of the pandemic, the sense of loss has been foregrounded and is all-pervading. Within the new parameters of a dangerous environment, and the ongoing exacerbation of existing systemic issues on marginalized peoples, there is a nuanced grief and loss that people are experiencing – both tangible and intangible. Loss of freedom, people, structure, predictability, housing, food security, community, traditions, coping mechanisms, safety, physical touch – the list could go on (Hyder, 2020). The daily news updates reporting on cases and deaths due to the pandemic – the ever-increasing numbers confronted each one of us with the reality of death and loss. Globally, as of 18 March 2022, there have been 464,809,377 confirmed cases of COVID-19, including 6,062,536 deaths, reported to WHO. Statisticians in the United States[1] tell us that for each death there are nine people immediately impacted (Verdery et al., 2020), and thus there could be 54,562,824 people who have lost a close family member to COVID and are bereaved and dealing directly with grief caused by the death of a loved one.[2]

Grief is universal and each one of us has and will experience loss as we go through the various attachments in life. It is sometimes experienced in its raw form, emanating from an explicit loss; at other times grief is experienced in subtle ways, maybe as a reflection of unmet desires. Suffering, loss, and grief are inevitable realities of human existence. Philosophers, artists, economists, and psychologists have all tried to approximate the texture and magnitude of loss and grief during the pandemic – a lot has been lost and we may not yet have even understood all that has been taken away.

Grief can be experienced and expressed in numerous ways – in thoughts, feelings, and emotions, and through bodily symptoms, it is a complex state and contains an amalgamation of many emotions such as denial, love, anger, sadness, betrayal, and the expressions of grief are variable. The constellation of grief is complex and is an area warranting extensive study. Grief is a complex emotion – usually understood as an expression of the experience of loss. We need to create a distinction between loss – the act of having to manage without something/someone who was important, close as well as loved and grief, the complex feeling emanating from that loss. Bereavement is understood in the context of the loss of a loved one. The expression of grief and the process of adapting to loss can vary dramatically from person to person, influenced as it is by the individual's own personality, temperament, beliefs, age, as also by culture, social practices, relationships, and so on.

The losses that the pandemic has thrown at us have been of various kinds. It is important in this context to understand non-finite losses – losses that are enduring in nature, usually precipitated by a negative life event or episode that retains a physical and/or psychological presence in an ongoing manner, leading to an ongoing sense of helplessness and powerlessness associated with the loss. Jones and Beck (2007) further add to this a sense of chronic despair and a sense of ongoing dread as the world view of individuals who have experienced grief becomes bleak and the future seems desolate. This sense of ongoing dread and of being suspended in an everlasting gloom of despair has been a common feeling pervading the pandemic. Chronic loss is best understood as a set of pervasive, profound, continuing, and recurring grief responses resulting from a significant loss or absence of crucial aspects of oneself (self-loss) or another living person (other-loss) to whom there is a deep attachment. The way in which the loss is perceived determines the existence of chronic sorrow. The essence of chronic sorrow is the painful discrepancy between what is perceived as reality and what continues to be desired. The loss is ongoing since it is experienced as a living, ever-present loss.

The pandemic also uncovered umpteen instances of ambiguous loss – losses that are difficult to name, describe, or validate – losses that cannot be explicitly defined. These unnamed losses create a sense of impending and continued grief, but since they remain unnamed, their acknowledgement and how to deal with them often elude us. Such losses may be experienced as irritability, have physical manifestations, and may continue to be evaded. The unending news of deaths and the despair caused by the untamable virus, which was also mutating and is continuing to produce new variants, contributes to the experience of anticipated loss. This is characterized as a sense of impending doom – a feeling that something/someone is set to be lost. We experienced an increase in the reporting of anxiety, depression, and paranoia; the sale of psychiatric medication increased. Shigemura et al. (2020) have pointed out that the pandemic lead to a sense of fear, anxiety, loneliness – to emotional outbursts and sleep disturbances. Issues with anxiety, sleep, stress, and suicide due to COVID-19 are also discussed by Sher (2020). The fear associated with infection and the anticipation of its severity and death contributed to feelings of impending doom and in more severe cases led to panic attacks, depression, paranoia, and suicide (Ornell et al., 2020). Such a widespread impact of COVID on mental health makes it imperative to explore its ramifications.

Theories of grief

Human existence is intertwined with experiences of grief, and theory continues to attempt to arrive at an accurate representation of the experience.

Authors and practitioners have proposed various theoretical approxima-
tions and best practices with which to address grief (Kubler-Ross, 1969;
Parkes, 1996; Rando, 1993; Stroebe & Schut, 1999; Worden, 2002). Existential thinkers provided insights into the inevitability of loss and suffering as existence is steeped in them. Grief is not a disease, but there is a
possibility that some people will become ill from grief. Freud's 'Mourning
and Melancholia' (1917/1955) includes a description of what normal and
abnormal grief are supposed to entail (Burstow, 1992). Freud pointed out
that grief can also be caused by the loss of fatherland, freedom, or an ideal.
He claimed that it is wrong to regard grief as pathological and something
requiring treatment. Grief passes after some time, and upsetting this process
unnecessarily may be harmful. By this, Freud perhaps meant that we should
trust the human ability to endure stress and strain and overcome hardship
through personal effort (Knutsen, 2020). Freud observed that the mourning
process can assume a pathological form if the relationship with the deceased
was overly characterized by ambivalent feelings and/or if the mourner had
a proclivity to 'narcissistic object-choice', that is, too many immature fea-
tures. A person can perceive an 'object loss' (such as bereavement) as an
injury to his or her ego. Freud believed further that the pre-condition for
this skewed personality development is frustration at the earliest stage of
life. It is implicit in Freud's text that mourning is a conscious as well as an
unconscious process, and that grief always encompasses multiple narratives.
In complicated mourning, the internal representations of the deceased (the
introject) do not merge with the mourner's self-representation, as in ordinary mourning (identification); they seem to continue having an independent experience (Volkan, 1970).

Freud has been widely read, studied, and also criticized for his views on
mourning and depression. Léon Wurmser (2015) expressed discomfort at
Freud's use of the terms 'object' and 'object loss' and stated that a person
to whom one is close cannot be an object, unless he or she is dehumanized (Knutsen, 2020). Instead of the concept of 'object loss', Kanwal (2016)
presents interpersonal approach to the understanding of grief and claims
that this is rather a matter of destabilization of a self-system that consists
of integrated interpersonal experiences. Finding 'new objects' is the same
as integrating new interpersonal experiences to re-stabilize this self-system.
Kanwal, who grew up in India, also emphasizes how the mourning process is linked to both, the cultural context around the mourner and the
circumstances that surrounded the bereavement in question. Also, Freud
missed addressing the growth opportunities that a completed mourning process entails, at an advanced age especially when loss is inevitable (Kernberg,
2010).

Modern psychoanalysis emphasizes the relational aspect, including when
it comes to the experience and processing of grief. Hagman claims that when
assessing the mourning process, we need to consider individual, familial,
and situationally dependent cultural and religious variables. The mourner

must find new roles and a new content in life (Hagman, 1995). According to Freud, he or she must gradually learn by reality orientation that the loved one is gone forever. Associations with the memories of this person must be dissolved and brought to a close, one by one. This is a painful process, and most people resist it for a while. When Freud lost his grandchild (Lieberman & Kramer, 2012), he felt that it destroyed something within him and made it difficult for him to establish emotional ties with others (Knutsen, 2020). Later, Freud stated that although it can be said that the acute mourning phase will pass, the sense of loss will remain, perhaps forever. Many stage- or phase-based models have emerged since Freud's, including Kubler-Ross's (1969) model for dying and bereavement, in which she argued that individuals follow a trajectory from stages of denial to acceptance. The five stages of grief include: denial, anger, bargaining, depression, and acceptance. Grief was seen to progress over these five stages on the continuum of time, establishing the role of spatial and temporal distance impacting the experience of grief. A passive engagement with grief may extend into immobilization at first and depression later. The phase model of bereavement, based on attachment theory, describes the process of grieving as consisting of four phases: the phase of numbing, the phase of yearning and searching, the phase of disorganization and despair, and the phase of reorganization (Bowlby, 1980). Parkes (1996) expanded Bowlby's model and conceptualized it as an individual moving through phases of numbness to recovery. He emphasized that grief was a psychological transition which changed our assumptive world.

The control and predictability that was assumed to be the order of the world was challenged during the pandemic – contributing to and being reflected in our grief responses. Worden (2002) offered a model in which one is given tasks to achieve, ranging from accepting the reality of one's loss to moving on with one's life. Rando's (1993) work in the area of complicated mourning includes three broad phases with many tasks to be accomplished before one can successfully grieve. Stroebe and Schut (1999) created a dual-process model in which individuals are seen as oscillating between a state of coping with practical aspects of bereavement and coping with the personal aspects of the loss. This theory presented two orientations within which individuals operate – loss orientation, which emphasizes the feelings of loss and yearning for the deceased and a restoration orientation, which centres on the grieving individuals re-establishing roles and activities they had prior to the death of their loved one. It could be argued that these theories demonstrate a wide variety of approaches to the understandings of grief. However, they have also been criticized since central to their approaches is an attempt to get to the essence of and define a universalized grief – a desire to have grief 'figured out' so that it can be better managed and controlled (Hadad, 2008).

Loss and grief are embedded in social and relational contexts, and dominant constructions of grief lack an acknowledgement of this variability

(Breen & O'Connor, 2007; Gilbert, 1996; Silver & Wortman, 1989). Within grief literature, there is a paradoxical trend of recognizing the variability that exists in the grieving process while also trying to define what constitutes 'normal' and 'abnormal' grief (Breen & O'Connor, 2007). While all traditional theoretical models of grief have the potential to become overly prescriptive, linear, and medicalized, the theories that discuss 'abnormal' and 'complicated' grief imply a predetermined definition of appropriate grief. More specifically, these theories place an emphasis on the individual to recover from loss in a predetermined manner. This is dangerous because it opens up the possibility for failure, as not everyone can or will 'recover' from loss, nor will they do so in a specific way. These models provide important insights into the grieving process that some people may experience but are still predominantly constructed through the medical model, often without critique. Theories steeped in positivist notions of linearity and reason have constructed a universalized experience of loss and grief. Yet, across these disciplines, grief has become a highly contested discursive terrain, affecting definitions, perceptions, and conceptualizations about what it means to experience loss. Dominant discourses on grief have made 'normal' the practices of pathologizing, othering, and essentializing those living with grief (Ord, 2009). These theories can help aid us in understanding the broad notions and processes in grief responses. However, what needs to be borne in mind at all times is that grief is complex and we need to allow individuals to take their path to express, experience, and integrate the loss.

It has been a little over two years since the pandemic and its massacre began. Our lives and our narratives have been altered forever – there is no going back to the world as we knew it. The experiences of losses – loss of autonomy, loss of the process and routine of life, loss of our older selves, financial losses, loss of loved ones, and so on – are all real and mounting. There is a wave of mental health disturbances brought on by the pandemic awaiting us. The kinds of complex grief responses that need particular attention are discussed in the following section.

1   Disenfranchised Grief: This kind is best captured in the inability to acknowledge and thus mourn the loss. The term disenfranchised grief was coined by Kenneth Doka, who defined it as the process in which the loss is felt as not being 'openly acknowledged, socially validated, or publicly mourned' (1989). This experience of grief could pose difficulties in terms of emotional processing and expression, as one may not recognize his/her right to grieve – in terms of social support, by diminishing the opportunity to freely express their emotions, and to obtain expressions of compassion and support. COVID-19-related deaths are in multiple ways lonely and dehumanized processes for patients and families. The pandemic has deprived the deceased of their dignity and has heightened the grief of those left behind (Pandey & Tripathi, 2021). Limitations in self-efficacy, choice, and control not only change the landscape of grief

and grieving but pose a significant risk and added burden in the already arduous and painful grieving experience (Albuquerque et al., 2021). The pandemic took away our cultural practices and made mourning an intensely individualized activity – sometimes painfully away even from the deceased. There have been numerous accounts of the bereaved not being able to see dear ones who had died or perform traditional rituals for them. Some lost parents while being in another country and couldn't come back to either tend to them when they were sick or perform religious rituals when they passed away; some were home with them a couple of weeks ago but didn't get to see their loved ones after they were hospitalized; some were sick themselves and couldn't be with even the closest family when one of them succumbed to COVID. All of these and many more are agonizing experiences of having 'suddenly' lost a loved one without a sense of closure. Rituals regarding the death and grieving process according to cultural practices have important functions (Burcu & Akalın, 2008). Albuquerque et al. (2021) identify therapeutic functions in the funeral rituals as they assist family members and friends in recognizing and confronting the reality of the loss, and offer room for introspection on death as a process integral to life and foster the awareness and assimilation of the grief process. These rituals help in the acceptance of the loss, providing emotional support, making it easier to express feelings and thoughts, and providing relief (Gross, 2016; Ozel & Ozkan, 2020). Funeral ceremonies bring people together to share memories of the deceased (Mallon, 2008). Rituals help people regain the sense of control and to cope with the grieving process (Norton & Gino, 2014). The pandemic took away the opportunity to perform these rituals and, more importantly, the continued isolation – even in moments of grief – impacted the grief response, mourning, and its reconciliation. There was no handing over of the dead bodies, no paying last respects, no rituals to bid farewell, no final goodbyes. This was further complicated by the fact that many of the deaths during the pandemic were sudden. The accumulation of death and loss in the larger reality may at first look as though it presents more opportunity to talk about, revisit, and share trauma, but the experience of increasing accumulation of deaths can also impede acknowledgement of each individual's grief. The deaths framed as statistics also leave bereaved individuals feeling that the pain of their loss in undervalued.

2   Complicated or prolonged grief: This is characterized by common grief reactions lasting for a longer time with unchanged, undiminished, or even increasing strength and frequently combined with self-reproach associated with the deceased person. The process of mourning fails or becomes prolonged such that the bereaved is unable to 'feel alive'. The loss of autonomy and helplessness at not being able to be with their loved ones during their last moments, sometimes after knowing that they will not make it out of the ICU alive, coupled with the inability to

perform the rituals that the dead 'deserved' led most of us to feel guilt. This is combined with the distressing feeling of having come out of the pandemic alive – leading to a feeling of survivor's guilt.

> Ray and Rosemary Scovell, from Sandown on the Isle of Wight, had been looking forward to their golden wedding anniversary when Ray, 76, fell ill. Their daughter Claire Apsey and grandson, Simon, said their grief had been compounded by lockdown. Mrs Apsey said she also felt 'guilty' for being unable to give them the send-off they deserved. . . . Although she was allowed to be with her father when he died, Mrs Apsey said she was 'gowned up' and had to wear a face shield. 'It wasn't the ending we wanted,' she said. A little over a week after losing her husband, Mrs Scovell ended up in hospital after a fall. X-rays revealed she had inflammation on her lungs and she tested positive for Covid-19. She died five days later. Mrs Apsey said: 'It's been horrific really. . . . The hardest thing is not being able to share the grief.'
>
> The funeral arrangements and contact with the solicitor, which had to be done via email, had also been 'so clinical', Mrs Apsey said. 'When we had my dad's funeral, I felt so guilty there were only 30 people there,' she added. 'It felt so wrong because my dad was so well known.' (BBC, 2021)

The complicated grief response may also include a sense of having lost part of oneself. The main feature that prevents grief from becoming pathological is the mourning process (Nakajima, 2018). Such a psycho-physiological process requires time, which is a critical and complex variable: clinicians assess not only the mere flow of time but also the subjective way this experience is lived. Failure to accomplish the integration of the deceased results in the so-called CG syndrome, where avoidance of grief, anger, guilt feelings, and reminders of death and loss have a key role as maintenance factors (Shear et al., 2011). Several variables (i.e., psychiatric comorbidities, nature of the relationship with the deceased, ways of coping with experienced mourning, family support) may affect the mourning process, making it different from one person to another. J. William Worden, a Harvard grief specialist, enumerates the important tasks of mourning to include acceptance of loss, acceptance of pain, adjustment to the new environment, and investment in the idea of starting a new life (Worden, 2002). The absence of mourning makes it difficult for people to come to terms with their loss. Also, the limited and sometimes no interaction with the world outside of one's home makes attempts at reconciliation with the loss difficult. It is important to distinguish this from depression. In depression, the awareness of loss is not so prominent, whereas in prolonged grief we can observe an intense and persistent longing for the deceased person. Symptoms of depression are more general and global, combined with brooding, dejection, and feelings of hopelessness.

3 Anticipatory Grief: The concept was proposed and theorized by Erich Lindemann (1944), characterized by acknowledging grief before the loss occurs. As opposed to grief occurring after the death of a loved one (referred to as *conventional grief*), anticipatory grief sets in during the time leading up to the anticipated passing away of a loved one, and the journey leading up to it can be a great deal more intense than the post-mortem path to recovery and healing. Those who go through the process of anticipatory grief are already trying to deal with the absence of a loved one – even with that loved one still by their side. This is bound to create an imbalance and dissonance and may give rise to feelings of guilt. Anticipatory grief is a multifaceted process and doesn't just have a focal point on a person's passing away. Dealing with anticipatory grief during the pandemic involved a sudden change in the roles fulfilled in the family, having to deal with the loss of dreams, dealing with the imminent loss of a loved one who may be infected and struggling, fears related to possible financial challenges, anger at the inability to help or save a loved one – complicated further during the second wave because of the burden on the ill-prepared medical infrastructure and lack of essentials needed for treatment such as the unavailability of oxygen cylinders leading to a feeling of acute helplessness.

Grief is not just a psychological issue experienced and expressed individually – it is influenced and shaped by cultural ideas, social values, fundamental assumptions, relational realities, and contextual vulnerabilities, so there needs to be a contextual understanding of loss and its expression.

Srikala is a commercial sex worker living in Mumbai's Kamatipura red-light area. She is middle-aged, short with a thick-set body. She is from Karnataka and came to live in Kamatipura some years ago. 'I am ugly, so I would not get a lot of clients. I would stand on the roadside near CST station and pick up clients there. On days I did not feel like travelling to CST, I would solicit clients in Kamatipura,' says Srikala. The minimum she charged from a client was Rs 150 for an hour of intimacy. On a 'good' day of business, Srikala earned Rs 1,000–1,500 a day. The years of the pandemic have taken their toll on her health and her finances. With no clients coming to her kholis (rooms), Srikala has plummeted into abject poverty. During the lockdown a few clients did brave the walk to the kholi, but the police clampdown scared even these few away. '*Daru ka dukaan bandh tha. Hamare paas shudhi mey kaun aayega, daru peekar aayega. Daru nahi dhandha nahi. Bheek maangke khate*' (The liquor shops were shut. No one comes to us in their senses, they come in an inebriated state. No liquor so no business. I beg for a meal), narrates Srikala. With no income, she plans to move out of Kamatipura and lose herself in the vastness of Mumbai.

(Deshpande, 2022)

While dealing with and exploring grief with a person going through loss, we must bear in mind the emotional state of the bereaved, economic realities, spiritual assumptions, interpersonal relations and social support, day-to-day changes, as well as physical expressions of grief. Loss and grief and making sense of oneself and the world thereafter are processes intertwined in the philosophical, psychological and physical realms of human existence and interaction.

COVID also saw a humanizing display of communities coming together to traverse and negotiate this individual and global crisis. During the second wave of COVID infections in India, communities emerged as resilient entities across the country. India's ethos, value systems, and cultural strengths automatically generated new energies and scores of new groups. Community action enabled society to overcome the failure of the state and the market (Chaturvedi, 2021). The idea of community coping and support networks made available opportunities for sharing – both the loss and resources that could help others. There were numerous social media accounts and channels providing medical support, arranging for beds at hospitals, providing food and medication, mobilizing relief activities, and working relentlessly to help fellow human beings in a crisis. This also became a space for catharsis and dealing with one's own loss(es) – it provided a sense of purpose, pride, and satisfaction as well as direction to the otherwise deleterious and pessimistic atmosphere.

Is there a thing as going back to normal? Are we changed forever? The overemphasis on coming back to 'normal' after the 'process of grieving' is perhaps a misnomer. Since there has been an experience of grief that has altered, perhaps in significant ways, the course of one's life and psychological realities, it needs to be borne in mind that this experience will continue to impact the individual and the entire community. Many lives have been altered forever – and there are non-finite losses that will be negotiated for a long time and will have an everlasting impact on the mourners. The process of mourning too was felt to be truncated – a loss was immediately followed by caregiver responsibilities towards the others in the family down with the illness – or caring for oneself through the onslaught of symptoms or of fear. It will be important to note the renegotiations and revisiting of the grief and mourning as people move back into some kind of 'normalcy' – the grief that they somehow accepted (or continued to deny) in their isolated existence will now have to be spoken about, shared and experienced all over again. The lives that were altered due to the pandemic had also cocooned the mourners from *normalcy*. A 24-year-old male student, who had lost his mother and uncle during the second wave, shared that he was feeling lost and was unable to negotiate reality as now he was expected to go back to living his pre-pandemic life – 'but it included my mother and I don't know what normal means without her'. A 9-year-old girl who lost her father in the second wave doesn't want to go to school anymore, even after they have reopened after two years, because she will 'miss papa more' when she comes back home to find it without her father. The pandemic has left many open wounds, and as the world tries to recover from the onslaught, the losses are and will become more real and glaring.

Integrating grief

As we take small steps towards regaining our lost social engagements and work commitments; as the world opens up allowing free movement and travel, we must acknowledge the change and make space for allowing the process of grief. We as a community need to be sensitive to the various forms grief may take – checking if there are physical symptoms that might need medical attention. Learning from the strength and resilience that community participation and integration brings, we need to organize our resources to build peer support networks. We may never be able to completely deal with this mammoth grief and its aftermath but a beginning can be made by 'sitting in', sharing, and listening. The idea here is to provide a holding space, bearing witness to the struggles and pain and being there. The focus is not on taking away the pain but respecting the processes and difficulties in the experience; not expecting an organized account of the event or the distress but allowing verbalizations regarding unfinished conversations, difficult parts of the relationship, and moving towards integration and acceptance. Work may not end in one span or a continuous block of time. Grief may come in waves. Some important events in life could be hard and may need emotional work and reconciliation. Presence and support of professionals wherever needed without pathologizing grief is a sensitive balance that needs to be maintained. It may be appropriate (and humane) not to think of grief counselling with a specific agenda of alleviating the grief but to support the bereaved individual in working out the process of grief in ways that are aligned with that person's values, view of himself/herself, personality, and temperament.

Notes

1 It is important to note that this is a study based in America; if a similar study is done in India the estimation of the direct impact of loss of a loved one may be much higher than 9:1.
2 According to newspaper reports, more than 25,000 children have lost a parent to COVID in the state of Maharashtra alone (Gangan, 2022).

References

Albuquerque, S., Teixeira, A. M., & Rocha, J. C. (2021). COVID-19 and disenfranchised grief. *Frontiers in Psychiatry*, *12*, 10–13. https://doi.org/10.3389/fpsyt.2021.638874
BBC. (2020, April 7). *Coronavirus: The world in lockdown in maps and charts.* www.bbc.com/news/world-52103747

BBC. (2021, February 27). *Covid: 'I lost both parents in two weeks'*. www.bbc.com/news/uk-england-hampshire-56182679

Bowlby, J. (1980). *Attachment and loss*. Basic Books.

Breen, L., & O'Connor, M. (2007). The fundamental paradox in the grief literature: A critical reflection. *Omega, 55*(3), 199–218.

Burcu, E., & Akalın, E. (2008). Sociological discussions of the death phenomenon. *Hacettepe University Turkic Studies, 8*, 29–54.

Burstow, B. (1992). *Radical feminist therapy: Working in the context of violence*. SAGE.

Chaturvedi, S. (2021, May 25). Why community efforts are essential for real change. *The Indian Express*. https://indianexpress.com/article/opinion/columns/second-wave-covid-infections-fcra-ngo-help-niti-aayog-7328874

Deshpande, H. (2022, February 11). Living on the edge: The pandemic and its axe on the migrant workers. *Outlook*. www.outlookindia.com/magazine/story/india-news-living-on-the-edge-the-pandemic-and-its-axe-on-the-migrant-workers/305411

Doka, K. (1989). *Disenfranchised grief: Recognizing hidden sorrow*. Lexington Books.

Freud, S. (1955). Mourning and melancholia. In *The standard edition of the complete psychological works of Sigmund Freud, vol. 14* (pp. 1957–1961). Hogarth Press (Original work published 1917).

Gangan, S. (2022, February 11). 25k children in Maharashtra have lost a parent to Covid. *The Hindustan Times*. www.hindustantimes.com/cities/mumbai-news/25k-children-in-maharashtra-have-lost-a-parent-to-covid-101644603405387.html

Gilbert, K. (1996). We've had the same loss, why don't we have the same grief? Loss and differential grief in families. *Death Studies, 20*(2), 269–283.

Gross, R. (2016). *Understanding grief: An introduction*. Routledge.

Hadad, M. (2008). *The ultimate challenge: Coping with death, dying and bereavement*. Nelson Education.

Hagman, G. (1995). Mourning: A review and reconsideration. *The International Journal of Psychoanalysis, 76*(Pt. 5), 909–925.

Hyder, S. (2020). COVID-19 and collective grief. *Child & Youth Services, 41*(3), 269–270. https://doi.org/10.1080/0145935X.2020.1834999

Jones, S. J., & Beck, E. (2007). Disenfranchised grief and nonfinite loss as experienced by the families of death row inmates. *Journal of Death and Dying, 54*(4), 281–299. https://doi.org/10.2190/A327-66K6-P362-6988

Kanwal, G. S. (2016). Death: The last chapter. In S. Akhtar & G. S. Kanwal (Eds.), *Bereavement. Personal experiences and clinical reflections* (pp. 169–190). Routledge.

Kernberg, O. (2010). Some observations on the process of mourning. *The International Journal of Psychoanalysis, 91*(3), 601–619. https://doi.org/10.1111/j.1745-8315.2010.00286.x

Knutsen, T. (2020, March). The dynamics of grief and melancholia. *Tidsskrift for den Norske Legeforening, 140*(5). https://doi.org/10.4045/tidsskr.19.0504

Kubler-Ross, E. (1969). *On death and dying*. Macmillan.

Lieberman, E. J., & Kramer, R. (2012). *The letters of Sigmund Freud & Otto Rank inside psychoanalysis*. Johns Hopkins Press.

Lindemann, E. (1944). Symptomatology and management of acute grief. *American Journal of Psychiatry, 101*, 141–148.

Mallon, B. (2008). *Dying, death and grief: Working with adult bereavement*. SAGE.

Nakajima, S. (2018). Complicated grief: Recent developments in diagnostic criteria and treatment. *Philosophical Transactions of the Royal Society of London: Series B, Biological Sciences, 373*(1754). https://doi.org/10.1098/rstb.2017.0273

Norton, M. I., & Gino, F. (2014). Rituals alleviate grieving for loved ones, lovers, and lotteries. *Journal of Experimental Psychology: General, 143*(1), 266–272.

Ord, R. L. (2009). 'IT'S LIKE A TATTOO': Rethinking dominant discourses on grief. *Canadian Social Work Review, 26*(2), 195–211. www.jstor.org/stable/41669912

Ornell, F., Schuch, J. B., Sordi, A. O., & Kessler, F. H. P. (2020). "Pandemic fear" and COVID-19: Mental health burden and strategies. *Brazilian Journal of Psychiatry, 42*(3), 232–235.

Ozel, Y., & Ozkan, B. (2020). Psychosocial approach to loss and mourning. *Current Approaches in Psychiatry, 12*(3), 352–367.

Pandey, A., & Tripathi, K. (2021). Death and dying during Covid- 19 pandemic: The Indian context. In P. Pentaris (Ed.), *Death, grief and loss in the context of COVID-19* (pp. 254–266). Routledge.

Parkes, C. (1996). *Bereavement: Studies in grief in adult life*. Taylor & Francis.

Rando, T. (1993). *Treatment of complicated mourning*. Research Press.

Shear, M. K., Simon, N., Wall, M., Zisook, S., Neimeyer, R., Duan, N., Reynolds, C., Lebowitz, B., Sung, S., Ghesquiere, A., Gorscak, B., Clayton, P., Ito, M., Nakajima, S., Konishi, T., Melhem, N., Meert, K., Sch, M., . . . Keshaviah, A. (2011). Complicated grief and related bereavement issues for DSM-5. *Depression and Anxiety, 28*(2), 103–117. https://doi.org/10.1002/da.20780

Sher, L. (2020). COVID-19, anxiety, sleep disturbances and suicide. *Sleep Medicine, 70*, 124. https://doi.org/10.1016/j.sleep.2020.04.019

Shigemura, J., Ursano, R. J., Morganstein, J. C., Kurosawa, M., & Benedek, D. M. (2020). Public responses to the novel 2019 coronavirus (2019 – nCoV): Mental health consequences and target populations. *Psychiatry and Clinical Neurosciences, 74*(4), 281–282. https://doi.org/10.1111/pcn.12988

Silver, R., & Wortman, C. (1989). The myths of coping with loss. *Journal of Consulting and Clinical Psychology, 57*, 349–357.

Stroebe, M., & Schut, H. (1999). The dual process model of coping with bereavement: Rationale and description. *Death Studies, 23*(3), 197–224. https://doi.org/10.1080/074811899201046

Verdery, A. M., Smith-Greenaway, E., Margolis, R., & Daw, J. (2020). Tracking the reach of COVID-19 kin loss with a bereavement multiplier applied to the United States. *Proceedings of the National Academy of Sciences of the United States of America, 117*(30), 17695–17701. https://doi.org/10.1073/pnas.2007476117

Volkan, V. (1970, December). Typical findings in pathological grief. *The Psychiatric Quarterly*, (44), 231–250. https://doi.org/10.1007/BF01562971

WHO. (2020). *Coronavirus (Covid-19) outbreak*. Springer. www.euro.who.int/en/health-CounsellingandGriefTherapy

Worden, J. W. (2002). *Grief counselling and grief therapy: A handbook for the mental health practitioner* (3rd Ed.). Springer.

Wurmser, L. (2015). Mourning, double reality, and the culture of remembering and forgiving: A very personal report. In L. W. A. Tutter (Ed.), *Grief and its transcendence: Memory, identity, creativity*. Routledge.

12 Living in the times of pandemic

Reliving and remembering loss and trauma

Shweta Dharamdasani

Present: October 2021

It has been one year and seven months since the first countrywide lockdown was imposed. A lot has changed since March 2020 and yet nothing has changed in many ways. We are still inside our homes, struggling to work from home and find a work-life balance. Masks and physical distancing have become a part of our social interactions. People are slowly and gradually returning to work. Some of us have learnt effective ways to work from home, while many are struggling to find work and survive. We have vaccines to provide some protection against the virus, yet people are suffering and dying. There are conversations about yet another wave and what that could look like. Each day feels easier and difficult at the same time, easier as the day passes by and difficult as with each passing day the reality of COVID continues to exist whether we acknowledge it or not. And what makes it harder are the multiple losses that each one of us continues to experience for the last one and a half years.

As a psychotherapist working in India, one is privy to socio-economic realities that govern our everyday reality. Health and sanitation facilities are grim. In a country where access to water to wash hands, and a piece of cloth to cover one's face, is a luxury, I wonder: how do we make sense of the numbers that the government puts forward to us while thinking about the impact of the virus? The sheer denial of the severity of the situation and the lack of resources on part of the government was at the heart of what India experienced in April 2021, when the second wave hit us. There was no day during that time that I didn't hear of someone in the circle who has either tested positive or lost a loved one. Losses were unbearable and too many. How do those who survived make sense of their feelings during the pandemic and the multiple losses that we all are experiencing? And not to forget about the post-COVID complications that follow recovery.

All this brought up some questions for me. Are we as individuals and community repressing feelings about loss? Are we repeating the same old treatment of our emotions? Or are we remembering and thus moving towards mourning and accepting the 'new normal'? What do our responses as individuals and as a group tell us about our individual and collective unconscious?

DOI: 10.4324/9781003255895-13

This chapter is an attempt at documentation of the ways in which we made sense and grappled with the wave of losses at the beginning of the pandemic.

The unconscious, it is said, is timeless. While practising psychoanalysis, one tries to make sense of the present through the past and vice versa. We try to do so through words. But how do we communicate our thoughts and feelings about loss? Do we have a language and vocabulary for it? Can words really capture the emotions evoked by an experience of loss?

This chapter is an invitation to the reader to make their own relationship with the text and find moments of the connection while reading. The chapter uses the personal, the social, and the clinical as three angles in understanding how big losses and everyday losses are intertwined with each other.

The chapter looks at the terms trauma and loss briefly from a psychoanalytic perspective. The first aperture to this exploration is my own response to the news of the death of two celebrities and my memories of my deceased grandfather, as the same day marked the six-month death anniversary of his. The news made me wonder about the process of mourning in the absence of rituals given the restrictions of curfew and physical distancing. The second aperture of my exploration becomes the collective response at a societal level. In order to do so, I look in detail at hoarding of toilet paper, excessive cooking, and so on as a way to deal with the anxiety that the pandemic has evoked in us, and what knowledge of the unconscious and defence mechanisms might have to offer in understanding human behaviour. A vignette from a case of a young woman with whom I have recently started working offers the third aperture in understanding the experience of loss and trauma. The vignette illustrates how the fear of losing a loved one to the virus brings back some unhealthy ways of relating and being in relationships due to unprocessed losses from the past.

Past: 12th May 2020

It is day 49 of the countrywide lockdown; lockdown 3.0. The total number of cases in India as of today is 70,756. While 22,455 people have recovered, 2293 people have lost their lives due to the virus. One doesn't have to be here for a webinar[1] to hear this. Why the webinar then? Why are we here as a community of mental health practitioners and students of psychology to discuss and think about loss and trauma? I will start by defining the two terms which are central to today's presentation and carry a lot of emotional charge: *loss* and *trauma*.

The Cambridge English dictionary defines loss as 'the fact that you no longer have something or have less of something'. In layman's terms, it simply implies the fact or process of losing something or someone. Psychoanalytically, loss can be understood as a loss of a breast, loss of faeces, or loss of an early love object (Freud, 1905/1964; Klein, 1935). For today's purpose, I would like to extend the same understanding and expand the meaning of loss. Loss is an experience that you no longer have something. And for the convenience of our understanding, let's divide it into two kinds: tangible loss and intangible loss. Loss of job, loss of money, salary cuts, and loss of a place to stay are examples of tangible losses. Loss of social interaction, not being able to go to work, and loss of sense of physical touch are examples of intangible losses. We are all together in this and it is something that we all are going through. Yes, we are together in this but does that mean we shouldn't be affected? Does the rule of majority work here too? Indeed, we can call it a collective loss, despite the pain and loss of each one having been affected individually as well,

And what about *trauma*? The word instantly evokes an experience of pain and sadness. Trauma is a severe and lasting emotional shock and pain caused by an extremely upsetting experience or a case of such shock happening. According to Sigmund Freud (1895as cited by Akhtar, 2009), 'any experience which calls up distressing affects – such as those of fright, anxiety, shame, or physical pain – may operate as a trauma'. As the psychoanalytic thought developed over time (Akhtar, 2009), trauma can be understood as a result of an internal and external event that stimulates the mind to an unbearable degree. Let's look at an example: someone who lost their job due to the crashing economy might start having self-deprecating thoughts such as 'I am not good enough' and may have bouts of sadness and anxiety. Now if one was to explore this, one can find long-standing patterns of thoughts and treatment of self which have always been there, lying around somewhere deep down in one's unconscious and it comes to the forefront as activated by an external event. Trauma then can be understood as any experience that creates a psychological injury.

Now after sorting out the defining business, the task at hand is, how do I talk about loss and trauma? In the last week, I kept thinking about the structure and the flow of the webinar and all my attempts went in vain. But wait! Aren't structure and well-articulated thoughts counter to the experience of loss? Do we have a language about and around loss? Maybe not, and as I was thinking the image of Amitabh Bachchan's tweet flashed.

'He's GONE . . .! Rishi Kapoor . . . gone . . . just passed away . . . I am destroyed!'

The words are there but the syntax of the tweet gives us a sense of rupture and disruption that trauma has on our psyche. Therefore, in an attempt to communicate my thoughts to you, this chapter is divided into three sections: the personal, the social, and the clinical. The three sections are three layers or angles through which I am making an attempt to think about what it is like emotionally to live in times of a pandemic.

The personal

It was 30 April when I was contacted to make a presentation in the webinar series. It was day 37 of the lockdown and I was in supervision at that time.

I was already feeling a little heavy that day as that very morning the news of Rishi Kapoor[2] succumbing to chronic illness came a day after Irrfan Khan's[3] demise. As uncanny as it may be but that day also marked six months of my grandfather's passing away. So when I got the call I asked for some more time. I wanted to think before I made any commitment.

The news, social media, and messages on WhatsApp were flooded about these two actors and their legacy and how they couldn't get the farewell they deserved. One of the dialogues that were making rounds everywhere was one from the movie *Life of Pi*: 'I suppose in the end, the whole of life becomes an act of letting go, but what always hurts the most is not taking a moment to say goodbye.' How did it sound so apt at the moment?

Feeling heavy in my chest and a sense of emptiness at the same time, I found myself thinking about this lockdown and the process of social distancing. Social distancing and lockdowns have limited access to chosen communities of close friends, siblings, and parental figures, and close friends. These relationships are critical in moderating our reactions to death (Mikulincer, 2018 as cited by Menzies et al., 2020). What did this do to our process of grieving and how does it impact our ability to mourn? How would it feel to not be able to see your father for the last time, to say goodbye and have closure? Visuals from my grandfather's funeral flashed. How difficult it would have been to bear the loss if the family hadn't been there. What would it be like if I didn't have my friends holding me when I was inconsolable? Culturally, 13-day rituals are deemed important as they allow us to mourn the loss. What do the absences of these rituals in the time of lockdown and restrictions do to the process of grieving and the experience of loss? Does it make it more lonely and painful? Or does it allow time and space to really sit with oneself and process the loss?

As I was sitting and listening to the news, my eyes welled up. I asked myself, what is happening? Yes, I was sad. I really liked both the actors and I know both of them were suffering from cancer. And maybe wherever they are they are hopefully at peace. So what was I feeling that made me teary? Without much struggle, I realized I was missing my grandfather and his presence. I thought I had mourned in some ways his absence as I have been open with friends and family about my feelings and also actively addressed them in my personal work. What is this lockdown and slowing of working hours doing to me? The fact that I am home, made me feel his absence more than ever in the last six months. After the first week of his passing away, I returned to work and got myself busy. That's how I dealt with it, to begin with. But now, it felt like there was another layer of grieving that needed to be attended to.

By absence, I do not mean just the physical absence of a body but the absence of the relationship, absence of conversations with him, seeing him around teasing my grandmother, hearing his thoughts on the pandemic, his life experiences. But all that I had was his empty room and the emptiness in my life. Was I alone in this? Surprisingly no. There were friends and family who shared that they too are going back to the memories of people who they have lost. And that there is something about the news of people dying and the sheer fear and dread the virus was triggering in all of us making us all feel so vulnerable that it was making us go back and remember our lost loved ones. But maybe this remembering and reliving are helping us re-work our way through the experience of loss, if not to at least acknowledge the loss. I allowed myself to sit there and cry.

The social

My interaction and observation of people around me and through social media confirmed my hypothesis that we as a society are terrible at talking and dealing with loss and complex emotions. We want to quickly get done with it. And fair enough. It is painful so let's brush it off under the carpet and bring out your armour of defence especially during a pandemic when the metaphor of war is used to fight a virus.

Isn't this what we are doing as a society? I mean technically we are living in a global pandemic that is here to stay for some time. The economy is crashing, people are dying, and children are not able to go to school or for outdoor play, no cricket, no music concert. It is SCARY!! This virus is like a *bin bulaya mehman jo apni marzi se aate hain apni marzi se jate hain* (an uninvited guest who comes and goes according to its own wish). Like good Indian hosts we serve them well, but is that what we feel within when someone uninvited comes to visit us? I doubt it. So let's look at what defences we as a society were using to deal with it. And when I say defence it is not necessarily pathological. All of us use defences in face of anxiety.

Let's start with the first big thing that was in the news after coronavirus: the hoarding of toilet paper (Ruane, 2020). Why would you want to hoard toilet paper and no other essential supplies? I mean literally, you won't poop if you don't have healthy food to eat. So, buy food and other essentials for which you may not have any other alternative. And how could I not go to Sigmund Freud (1905/1964) to understand this hoarding? The anal stage[4] according to Freud (1905/1964) is about learning control and letting go. So what is this act of hoarding toilet paper saying about the stuff under the carpet? I wonder if the lack of control that the pandemic brought with itself triggered some issues about control. It is like if I have things to keep myself clean I will have other things in control too. Interesting, huh!! This is a hypothesis about the West.

How are we Indians dealing with this? Are we different in dealing with the virus? May be yes! All my feeds on Facebook and Instagram and even some family groups are all about food recipes.[5] It seems as though everyone is competing in the master chef challenge but with their own self. Each day is a challenge to beat your own cooking skills from yesterday. Should we go to Sigmund Freud and see what he has to offer, or may be this time to Melanie Klein (1932) or Erik Erikson (1950) or maybe a platter of all three?

It is in the early years that we take in the world through the oral cavity and the pleasure we seek. It is not just the pleasure but also a relationship that the infant builds with the world outside and learns to trust or not trust the world for meeting his or her needs. Does the amount of food that has been made and the need to cook something new every day say something about what is under the carpet there? Maybe if we eat good tasty nutritious food we may start feeling differently about the world outside and within. Also, cooking as a process helps to release tension from the body. Therefore, some people find cooking really cathartic.

But what are we doing with images of a pregnant migrant woman walking thousands of kilometres to reach her safe space, and the news of 15 migrants who were run over by a train?[6] Are we, in our attempt to upgrade ourselves with each extended lockdown, trying to find external ways to control and keep alive a better and a fuller image of the world inside? Maybe yes. It is as though something inside us breaks and we build something.

But all the ways that we are coming up to deal with this new reality are not unhealthy. The lockdown has made us all realize our need for social interaction. Hence we have also had glimpses of how, when faced with a crisis, humans come up with the most creative ideas. We all know about balcony concerts in Italy. And then there were these videos of people playing *tambola* and people playing *bhajans* from their balcony to recent videos on TikTok of cleaning the house and sharing it virtually with each other. What are we trying to do? Entertain ourselves, yes, but also keep whatever sense of community we can, and that's wonderful.

This chapter, too, is part of an attempt to not feel the loss of community and to keep the connection alive. It may also be a need to feel that we are doing something to contribute to society in fighting the virus, which has probably now started to enter our minds in terms of fear and frustration. Therefore, we are trying to control the body through the mind, but as they say, something is better than nothing.

So far, we looked at how loss and trauma resurfaced from my personal experience of remembering my grandfather's demise triggered by the death of two celebrities and the absence of rituals and what they do to the process of mourning. And how the society as a whole is fighting the war against this virus on the outside and what it may mean on the inside. Now let's look at how the pandemic is entering into the 'clinic' and how the virtual medium is affecting the clinical work done given the current circumstances.

The clinical: 'Unfinished business of bereavement'

The clinic is often an appropriate reflection of what goes on in the world around us. As soon as the lockdown was imposed, the demand for mental health practitioners suddenly saw a rise. There was a palpable tension about what this lockdown was about to do with the range of emotional reactions/ feelings with which all of us were closed in our houses. What comes now is a vignette from the very early days of work with a client (who I continue to work with).

D, a 24-year-old female, first met me just five days before the countrywide lockdown was imposed. She contacted me as she was experiencing extreme anxiety and had suicidal thoughts. D came with a long-standing history of losses and unfinished business of bereavement. From the very first session, it was clear to me that this is a long-term work and may require bi-weekly sessions in person. When the lockdown was imposed, she decided to wait for three weeks and come in person, but who knew that the initial three-week lockdown was to be turned into a longer lockdown? With apprehension, we started the work online. The following sessions shed light on the unprocessed feelings of anger and sadness that were under all the anxiety.

D lives with her parents. She had two brothers, one younger and the other elder, both of whom passed away. The younger one succumbed to a medical condition early in his life. There is guilt in her when she talks about the younger one. She was two and a half years old when he was born, and since he used to be unwell and needed more attention at that time, she recalled having anger towards him for being there. She recalled how her mother had shared about the way D would sometimes look at him in anger. Just like in a two-and-a-half-year-old's internal omnipotent imaginative world, her anger might have killed him, which turned into guilt and now presents itself as a symptom of anxiety whenever she experiences anger towards someone she loves.

The other brother met with a road accident and couldn't survive the injury. She was close to the elder one. She shared how she was really upset (accessing anger at that point of time in our work was not possible for her: she was not allowed to be angry) when she realized that the family cremated her elder brother while she was asked to go and sleep and she could never say goodbye to him and see him for the last time. The family's explanation was that it would have been too painful for her to see. In our work, we explored how much anger there is underneath the pain of the loss of a sibling. The anger is also because of the family deciding what would be less painful for her. Sometimes in order to protect our loved ones from pain, we do more damage than good. Goodbyes are painful, but not having closure is far more painful. Saying goodbye and having to give words to an otherwise difficult experience help in resolution. The act/ritual of goodbye is crucial to the process of separation and loss and also to value the relationship that once existed. Endings matter and that is what stays with us as experiences.

Both her parents were working and now retired so all these years while growing up she was really close to her grandfather, who too passed away due to age-related health issues. Her mother was diagnosed with breast cancer a few years ago. Too much to even hear, right?

Apart from these repeated losses which had an impact on having a stable engaging love object while growing up, she had great difficulty at school, particularly with teachers. In short, one could say that D experienced adults as unloving, angry, ignorant of her feelings and thoughts, and reprimanding. Also due to these repeated losses and experiences in school, she started to believe that people leave because she is not 'good enough' or she is not a 'good girl'.[7] This had a huge role to play in her feeling anxious and wanting to die in face of difficult, complex emotions.

With the lockdown in place and not being able to meet some of her friends and talk to them in person who were her safe zone, she started to feel lonely, anxious, and sad. In a particular session, she was really disturbed as her ex-boyfriend's father was found to be coronavirus positive. She was scared and afraid that he too might be tested positive. The unknowability and the uncertainty of when she would get to see him were making her feel really anxious. The relationship that she was in had its own conflicts. However, as the work happened the unequal dynamic of their relationship became apparent. At the same time in therapy, we were talking about her feelings about the equation. This was new for her, as over the years she had learnt to take a backseat in relationships and let the other person's needs be at the forefront, so that the person does not leave her. She was assigned the role of attending to others around her from an early age when her brother passed away. She was told by her relatives that she needed to be strong as she needed to take care of her grieving parents, but what about her own grief? With these experiences in the background, the news of her ex-boyfriend possibly being infected with the virus not only triggered the fear of loss but also made her go to an earlier pattern of relating where she became the caregiver and neglected herself. For her, the fear of losing a relationship was far more painful and damaging than what an unequal relationship was doing to her. That session and the one after that were filled with her feeling anxious, manifesting itself in nightmares, headaches, and inability to sleep and eat.

These experiences of people leaving had a huge impact on our working relationship too. She would often feel that she is too much for me and that I might leave her. All of this was a projection from her past experiences. These past experiences acted as barriers when I was paying attention to her in the therapeutic relationship. The newness of this kind of exclusive engaging attention was scary and satisfying at the same time. The conflict of wanting to be attended to and not wanting the attention as it was unfamiliar would lead to her shutting down in sessions (yawning, dizziness, nausea) to avoid the experience of having to emotionally depend on therapy. Another way this would play out in our interaction was that she focused on others in her session and avoided talking about herself in therapy. Unconsciously, she wanted me to ask her to take care of herself and be an active participant in attending to her whereas she would continue to focus on others around her. Can my wish or need for her to grieve, bring any change in her capacity to actively participate in her life? Probably not. What is this helplessness? Is it part of her being? Yes. Or is helplessness also part of our collective response and specifically in her case reaction to a situation of crisis? Probably this too. The work with her since then has been around and about losses (in the last year and a half she lost her maternal grandfather, an aunt, a cousin, and a classmate) and making sense of these sudden losses and absences.

Don't we all feel helpless in situations where clearly the enemy is invisible? Is this the reason why the number of professionals offering counselling has suddenly gone up? There is a kind of mobilization in the field of psychology, psychiatry, and social work to fight this virus. Is that because we know at least theoretically the repercussion of such life-altering events?

But are we as psychologists/psychotherapists going to fight this battle having the right tool kit? I would suggest not. The temptation and the altruism in all of us would force us to take this task up of helping anybody who asks for it. But I will lay out my cautionary cards. In my experience, working on the screen brings along with it a lot of barriers. First, the screen is already a barrier between you and the client. It only increases the resistance in some clients by tenfold, which makes it far more difficult to work. Second, my personal experience says that it is never just coronavirus anxiety. It has to have deeper unconscious layers and usually, the calls that I have received in recent times are anxiety discharge calls. I have received messages at midnight asking if I am working online and if I have a slot. As soon as I reply, the person on the other side is gone.

Therefore, the link between and the internal and the external becomes crucial in understanding the impact of the pandemic on our psyche.

Tips to attend to oneself in the midst of chaos

As we reach the end of the chapter, it is no news that the virus affects not just our body but the mind too. The notion that our mind and body are connected is well known and accepted, whether you see this from a psychological viewpoint or the Indian notion of chakras. Now the challenge is how to build psychological immunity to protect your minds. By now you all must have found your own ways and what I will be sharing now might be a repetition. But repetition is a reminder.

1   To begin with, have a routine. It is very important to have a structure to the day especially when everything around seems to be falling apart and going haywire. It will add a sense of rhythm to our day and give us a sense of control at least in one's own life.
2   Find your social support group and reach out to them. It is really important to stay connected with friends and family, and to keep a check on them, especially in cases where home might not be the safest place one can be in. Use technology and various media to stay connected. However, keep a check on the usage of technology. It can become an added self-imposed layer to distancing, even while being in the same house. Therefore, a check on time spent on virtual media and apps is a must. If we are lucky enough to be around people who we love and feel safe with, the physical expression of affection such as hugs would be a great

way to cope with the level of distress and fear. Touch, as we know, helps restore us to health the fastest.[8]

3   The anxiety about the situation is real and can manifest itself in insomnia, restlessness, and being fidgety. Anxiety is experienced in the body and produces a kind of pressure that needs to be released. Some amount of physical activity and movement in the day will help to reduce anxiety. The activity could range from workouts to yoga to skipping a rope – anything that is doable. If it becomes unbearable reach out to a professional.

4   Most of us have hectic schedules outside this crisis and often leave no window to do something fun and creative. Here is the time. Find your hidden talent or revive the one that you have. Having created something helps us to hang in there and gives us hope; however, don't turn yourself into a project. Taking a day at a time is okay.

Postscript: Denial and the 'new normal'

The larger part of this chapter was written back in May 2020, at the very beginning of the pandemic. Some parts of the chapter still hold as true as they did back then, and there are some additions. What has been consistent is the denial of the reality and gravity of the situation. The idea of 'new normal' is being sold to us as a fancy package without any conversation about and around all that all of us have lost since the beginning of this pandemic. What does this 'new normal' mean to us and how does it impact us? The number of people on the streets without masks is scary.

The repetitive narrative that we have overcome the virus is of concern. We are letting our guard down, which did cost us a lot as a country during the second wave. There have been too many distractions to keep the disaster unseen and unnoticed whether it has been the economy plummeting or political upheavals or celebration of the number of vaccinations. However, it seems as if all of us have repressed what happened in April 2021 as an unpleasant memory and moved on.

One can only hope that this repressed virus does not come back in uglier forms like repressed feelings.

Notes

1   This chapter was presented in the form of a webinar at a series of webinars held by Bharati College, Delhi University, in May 2020. The series was aimed to initiate a conversation around mental health issues during the pandemic. The webinar took place in the relatively early days of this ongoing pandemic.
2   Indian actor, active in Hindi films from the 1970s until his death.
3   Indian actor, known worldwide for his art.
4   Freud (1905) gave five psychosexual stages of development. He believed that all of us are born with a pleasure seeking drive. He proposed that a child goes through various stages of development each with its erogenous zone. The anal stage is second in the chronology of stages. It starts from the age of one and goes up to three

years of age. The erogenous zone in this stage is the anus. The child seeks pleasure either by holding the faeces or releasing them. Toilet training is a very important aspect of this stage. The experience of toilet training in many ways defines the personality of the young adult. Being compulsive or being messy could be the two extreme outcomes.

5 See, for example, Akolawala (2020), Borah (2020) and '8 Most Popular Dishes' (2020).
6 This was reported in various newspapers and media. See, for example, Chaturvedi (2020).
7 A good girl is said to be who follows what is expected of her, who does not challenge the roles set for her by others, someone who is submissive (Dharamdasani, 2019).
8 See, for example, Cassata (2018).

References

8 most popular dishes during the lockdown. (2020, December 30). *The Times of India.* https://timesofindia.indiatimes.com/life-style/food-news/8-most-popular-dishes-during-the-lockdown/photostory/80013597.cms

Akhtar, S. (2009). *Comprehensive dictionary of psychoanalysis.* Karnac.

Akolawala, T. (2020, May 5). Top 5 most popular cooking apps downloaded during lockdown in India. *NDTV Gadgets 360.* https://gadgets.ndtv.com/apps/features/top-cooking-apps-android-google-play-apple-app-store-tasty-archanas-kitchen-yummly-tarla-dalal-recipes-2223899

Borah, P. M. (2020, August 11). Mission: Lockdown cooking. *The Hindu.* www.thehindu.com/life-and-style/food/lockdown-cooking-solutions-online/article32316311.ece

Cassata, C. (2018, June 27). How touching your partner can make both of you healthier. *Healthline.* www.healthline.com/health-news/how-touching-your-partner-can-make-both-of-you-healthier

Chaturvedi, A. (2020, May 8). Tired migrants sat on tracks for rest, fell asleep. 16 run over by train. *Hindustan Times.* www.hindustantimes.com/india-news/14-migrant-workers-mowed-down-by-goods-train-in-maharashtra/story-Z6V8QkOY2CGvdKNHv2uPvI.html

Dharamdasani, S. (2019). The work of secret – 'Desire among siblings'. Unpublished MPhil thesis. School of Human Studies, Ambedkar University Delhi.

Erikson, E. H. (1950). *Childhood and society.* W. W. Norton.

Freud, S. (1964). Three essays on the theory of sexuality. In J. Strachey (Ed.), *The standard edition of the complete psychological works of Sigmund Freud* (pp. 123–243). Macmillan. (Original work published 1905)

Klein, M. (1932). *The psycho-analysis of children.* Hogarth Press.

Klein, M. (1935). A contribution to the psychogenesis of manic-depressive states. *International Journal of Psycho-Analysis, 16,* 145–174. www.pep-web.org/document.php?id=ijp.016.0145a&type=hitlist

Menzies, R. E., Neimeyer, R. A., & Menzies, R. G. (2020). Death anxiety, loss and grief in the time of COVID-19. *Behaviour Change, 37*(3), 111–115. https://doi.org/10.1017/bec.2020.10

Ruane, M. E. (2020, March 18). Toilet paper takes center stage amid coronavirus outbreak. Be thankful we no longer use corn cobs and rope ends. *Washington Post.* www.washingtonpost.com/history/2020/03/18/toilet-paper-takes-center-stage-amid-coronavirus-outbreak-be-thankful-we-no-longer-use-corn-cobs-rope-ends/

13 Stairs and waves

On the shores of 'social' distancing

Ananya Kushwaha

Distance and contact: Introduction

In the pandemic the term 'social distancing' became very prevalent. First as an accepted form of 'breaking the chain' of infection', then as an aberration when people realised that one needn't isolate 'socially', but only 'physically'. Moreover, it dawned upon us that the 'social distancing' is likely to create further discrimination of already marginalised communities. The term was revised to 'physical distancing'. In its Hindi translations some airports and public areas corrected 'सामाजिक दूरी *(Samajik Doori* – social/community distancing) to 'शारीरिक दूरी (*Sharirik doori* – bodily distancing) while many places continued with a literal translation irrespective. What is striking is that even in Hindi the difference took quite a while to emerge and be marked while the meaning and its implications appear starker in the Hindi version indicating a sense closer to 'community' than just 'social'.

There is something important about literal translations and concreteness. The human mind is not built only for concreteness. Cognitive development theories mark the importance of the developmental achievement of symbolisation and abstract thinking by adulthood. The human mind is built for relational expansion so much so that a great part of our own words and worlds and their emotional meanings are expressed but unknown to our own selves and have an emergent quality – a discovery formalised and theorised by the advent of psychoanalysis (but familiar to the artists, poets, writers, dancers, musicians, lovers and creators and players).

Words carry a slice of the dynamic world around us and inside us because they transport meaning.[1] Our speech (written or oral) and our body are the two mediums through which we expand ourselves outwards and carry more than what we consciously intend to carry. As we recently discovered in the pandemic, our unselfconscious ways of being can transport and spread viruses! The times we live in and our cultural contexts also structure this expansion and constriction – one such example is our movement and its restriction as physically experienced in the lockdown due to the pandemic. In the late twentieth century, many of us grew up with aspirations of modernity, liberalism, education, independence, freedom to make personal choices

DOI: 10.4324/9781003255895-14

in love and career, and ideals of equality allowing for greater self-expressions. In India, a cultural shift took place over the past few decades in the direction of focus on 'self' and freedom for that discovery and expression. It may have overlapped with the zeitgeist. Most psychoanalytical therapists and psychologists in general will affirm that the referrals they have received are likely to have significantly increased over this last decade or so. However, many people will corroborate that their aspirations and ideals from their childhood and adolescence about the future and the situation in current times in which we live are very different. The simple 'middle-class' dream, which was also the dream for most upwardly mobile classes – a dream of good education, jobs, financial independence for women, more space for pleasure and aesthetics in life than just duties and toil which previous generations may have faced, is not simple anymore. Major shifts have happened at a fast pace in the social-political climate globally alongside a boom of virtual space and social media. Often termed as 'post-truth' in these times, a focus on political image management through marketing, polarising propaganda and segregation is at an all-time high. The political agendas have shifted from providing services to better the quality of life in terms of aspirations of education, healthcare, infrastructure and so on to intensification of an identity-based politics. Personal and social locations marked with caste, class, religious identity, gender identity as well as regional identity, such as hill dwellers, plains dwellers, refugees, migrants, local people and tribals, are some of the axes along which identity issues have always created marginalisation but have recently become central points of exclusionary politics.

It may be worthwhile to study the reasons for this shift over the last few decades in the socio-political situation with an odd mix of consumerist capitalism, global politics and social media and its impact on our subjectivity in these times. However, that is beyond the scope of this chapter. This is not about creating nostalgia for some great times lost in the past. While different aspects of changes in current times may be actually great in terms of awareness and global connection, the divides in their wake are humongous, and it is worth asking who and what gets left behind. This also has implications for what aspects of our speech and movement will be allowed and those that will be forced to be constricted and repressed (such as what will get spoken only in muted tones and in limited spaces as perhaps this chapter). It defines the narrowing limits of our 'freedom of speech' and democratic ideals because the space of speaking and listening is increasingly narrowing in the social sphere.

Phyllis Beren and Sheldon Bach's recent work 'Psychic Space' highlights another aspect of our times. They highlight how in the zeitgeist of our times the psychic and the physical spaces are continuously suffering an onslaught and constriction. They highlight the impact of sensationalism and social media and spread of polarising misinformation (Beren & Bach, 2018). One can say that news has become some perverted form of NEWS – too much new! Everything is being rendered new and isolated. 'Breaking news' is more like 'broken news' with no connection with larger contexts. Everything is a 'byte' – a small packet of sensational narratives, evoking things against your permission and wishes – an assault on the sensations, creating an overwhelming effect. The sensationalistic energy is in the air. It has become 'air-borne'. We are surrounded at all times by drones, cameras, chatting applications collecting data – 'personal' data. The line between personal and public is diffused. This results in 'instant' (in the age of instant messaging) alienation from our space to be ourselves, to reflect and to be creative. The authors in 'Psychic Space' talk about how this kind of an onslaught on the senses pulls us into a vortex of only responding and reacting to what we are fed, taking away an important transitional space[2] required for creativity and change from the status quo.

What is important to note through all this is that something about our subjectivity is at stake. Something about our 'democratic ideals' is at stake here, and it is of concern for the psychoanalytic community globally. The 'virtual couch' in the title of the book can also be thought of as a metaphor of our 'virtual' subjectivity as it emerges on the psychoanalytic horizon. Even as psychoanalysis went 'online' during this time, here I am also talking about a simulated identity proliferating in these times – more captured and projected in elements of data through software which gathers one's algo-rithms than actual presence. Can we say that the era of bodies and embod-ied minds is a thing of the past? 'Body', a personally belonging concrete sense of self embodied by one's desires as one discovers them over the life span, seems like an afterthought in this day and age, after the 'social' and 'media' (carrying forward the metaphor of social distance, physical distance and bodily distance[3]). Due to lesser psychic space available, the fixation on the 'imagery' and preoccupation with the Other's gaze, the embodied self is less an agentic self and more like a submission to the demands of the forces of sensationalism. The pandemic has precipitated and widened these fault lines in a way to a huge degree socially as well as at an individual level. One can say that the pandemic has highlighted and exaggerated our existing mental lockdown and isolation situation, our 'distancing' from 'contact' of any kind through its imperative of 'bodily distancing'. This chapter is an attempt to reclaim some in-between spaces – the space between words and their meanings, space between propaganda and facts, space between personal and social, space between 'contact' and 'distance', the space where psychoanalysts work – 'The Virtual Couch'.

The Indian scene: Stairs, stares and stars

If we looked at the evolution of some of the words over the past two years of the pandemic, we would realise what a journey they have been on. From 'social' first when 'contact' with others itself suddenly appeared as danger-ous and fatal, then as the fears about the spread of the virus and familiarity with it made it conceivable, it was re-calibrated as 'physical' and 'bodily'. At the same time, if we look at the public spaces and social landscape of India, as well as personal spaces, mostly words like 'masses', 'community' and 'crowd' carry with them important images and experiences of daily life. People are mostly squished body against body, bumper to bumper, in long lines, in constricted spaces. In such spaces, where is the possibility of 'distancing'? The distancing in the mind is a greater possibility than distancing of the body in a country like ours. No wonder, many times people stopped even making eye 'contact' during the initial days of the pandemic due to the fear of contagion. Not only that, but socially, the contagion was easily projected on certain social categories of people as 'carriers' of the virus, even though there was no rational and scientific reason to do so.

So deep is the social segregation and the stratification in our country that even doctors were heard subscribing to these attitudes of blaming specific communities for the spread of the virus. Meanwhile, paradoxes also emerged (luckily), challenging this discrimination. So even though poor people are often targeted as being blamed for living in congested areas with poor sanitation and therefore associated with spreading disease (even though these may be outcomes of systemic failures), this time actually those who could travel abroad became the first carriers of the disease – the 'patient zeros'. This virus spread among the rich as well as the poor irrespective, as long as people met and came in contact with other people (of course different vulnerabilities present other challenges of accessing healthcare, physical distancing, lack of income during lockdowns etc.). Yet, if the 'patient zero' was closer to a position of marginalisation and lack (zero), then their community would be blamed as disease carriers but if the 'patient zero' was closer to a secure social location, they were likely to be seen merely as medical patients. To what extent one is seen as an individual, and to what extent, as a member of a specific community, their identities restricted and constricted, depends on these social hierarchies. Individual voice is a privilege. To speak a personal tongue and speak for yourself is also a privilege now. People are rarely seen as 'persons' in the public domain and mostly as representations of parts of their social identity or political preference, irrespective of whether they identify with those representations or not. Where one is located on the identity ladder (stairs) structures how one will speak and be spoken about.

This is interesting because now your image as seen by others has become more relevant and 'real' than how you think about yourself. Jill Gentile's work is crucial in linking psychoanalytically notions of agency, democracy, the position of the third versus perversity of twoness (locked in fixation rather than symbolic freedom). In her work titled *Between Private and Public: Towards a Conception of the Transitional Subject*, she talks about how the importance of an outward expression of oneself as a symbol is a crucial aspect of development of our subjectivity. This requires an expression of our authentic self in the world and having a recognition of it in the interpersonal space. This enables individuals to also contribute to their social presence:

> [E]volution of subjectivity in which we create ourselves between subjectivity and materiality, private and public. In this process, we not only

contribute to material and cultural life through the creation of symbols (for example, the transitional object), but we actually create ourselves as symbols, becoming part of material and cultural life.

(Gentile, 2008, p. 960)

It is important to think about the outcome of a reverse possibility in the social space in which there is restriction and limiting of people's expressions in a way that it only matches a specific agenda. This kind of segregation creates a certain pull and urgency motivated by sensationalism and propaganda to fix images, meanings and sounds in the social-cultural sphere. It has created a buzzing noise ensuring no one listens and therefore no one speaks in this context. Speeches without an audience – without anyone receiving the speech/expressions. Blames, segregation and shaming aimed to further quieten any voices of difference or really any voices at all. The troll army in virtual space spreads like a virus, irrespective of who is speaking what, and infects and concretises all meaning, taking over the 'host' to serve a very specific function of exalting the cause of authoritarianism. Not to mention that there is a widespread presence of bots now in virtual space who just add 'keywords' enough to start a troll campaign. If we focus on these words and their sense, they capture a sense of invasion, cancellation, producing feelings of paranoia, fear, helplessness and self-consciousness and hyper-vigilance. Pretty much similar to the fear of contagion produced by COVID-19 virus.

India is called the largest democracy in the world. Again, let those words sway in your mind – (1) 'largest' and (2) 'democracy'. Personal space is a luxury available to very few, very privileged. One can only imagine what that means for personal voice, personal choice and expression. Whether it is owning a piece of land, having a room of your own, having access to some greenery or clean air, none of these things are equally available to all. On the one hand in India, the terms we associate with our surroundings are 'dirty', 'chaotic', 'broken system', 'crowds', 'people', 'poverty', 'hierarchy', 'lack of education' and, on the other hand, we also take pride in 'richness', 'diversity', 'community', 'blending' and so on. In such a system 'large' and 'democracy' if placed together are like two magnets with the same poles facing each other. The availability of 'free voice' of participation (as is the aspiration of democratic values) to such a large population especially collapsing from time to time in a majority-based politics rather than participatory politics is a much distant dream. Recently, around the time that the pandemic was just starting a top bureaucrat proclaimed that there is 'too much democracy'. As the second most populated country in the world, any organising principle imposed, even of the most authoritarian of regimes, is bound to burst at the seams.

This tension between excess (too much) and lack (limits) is an interesting subject for psychoanalysis. Psychoanalysis was born trying to make sense of that which did not fit in any existing frame of knowledge about our mental life. Our knowledge about our mind was limited to conscious and rational subjectivity. The 'excess' was not engaged with. A hysterical patient was not of much interest for the doctors beyond an establishment of the fact that physical symptoms could have no physiological underpinning until Freud and his patients decided to 'talk freely'. It wasn't the talking only (the speech) but the 'freely talking' – free association – because it opened up the dynamic nature of words and their meanings and the ways in which our mind uses symbolisation. It was an offer of space to speak freely which opened a new paradigm about our minds and a new way of knowing what is unknown, unformulated and uncertain. This was precisely because it suspended the fixation of meaning in the usual established forms and opened a possibility for going beyond that – beyond what was fixed and understood and established.

As a species, we human beings essentially relate with each other and the world around us through our bodies and language and symbolic expressions which are structured less like dictionary meaning and more like a 'sample' extract of the socio-cultural and individual's emotional experiences and lived realities. While the medically known notion of bodies and viruses will function as per the scientific logic, the experiences as expressed in our fantasies and emotional expressions capture another kind of reality of our social situation and location (the pre-existing fracture lines of our social systems). These experiences actually remain a source of all action despite our rational knowledge systems, so much so that when words fail, bodies move, and when bodies are restricted, the mind flies. Even though it may be harder to listen to personal tales beyond the identities fixed by the stares of those in power, like twinkling stars, the light emitted by the silences and silencing of that which is uncontainable will travel long and far even if reaching the eyes of the beholder only several years later. In the pandemic, the tales of migrant labourers in India, those from the 'unorganised' workforce, travelling thousands of kilometres for several days to deal with the sudden imposition of lockdown are one such example.

Unorganised

For many of us in Delhi, the pandemic struck at a time when recently many social upheavals had taken place over the course of 2019. Citizenship Amendment Act (CAA), an act which is now a law granting citizenship rights to refugees of certain religions but not to those of others), led to massive protests in different parts of the country. In December 2019 university students were beaten up and universities entered into by police, and then, as protests gathered further steam, and the political charge rose between opposing groups, violence erupted in north-east Delhi in February 2020. Houses were burnt in a wave of terror lasting a few days. Many were killed in the national capital of India. As relief was being mobilised to help the victims, the pandemic struck India in March 2020, and there was a nationwide lockdown announced towards the end of March within a matter of hours. One can say that the hate 'waves' and heat 'waves' and pandemic 'waves' were all rising away simultaneously. Migrant labourers started walking home in multitudes on foot. For many of us, it was a sudden awakening to the realisation that several people on whom we depend for various services like vegetable sellers, hawkers, construction labourers, house painters, house maids and so on have been migrants and living in dire conditions in the cities. This group is recognised as the unorganised[4] sector by the government and comprises 80–90 per cent of India's workforce. When the lockdown was imposed at very short notice, the migrants emerged like an afterthought to remind us that not everyone can afford to be in an unplanned lockdown. In multitudes, people started walking to their homes thousands of kilometres away. They walked for days.

In this climate some of us with backgrounds in psychoanalysis, development studies and social work came together to build an organisation called Zeest – Centre for Psycho-Societal Innovation. Zeest is formed to address the need to study and use psychoanalysis and its tools and techniques for better engagement strategies in the community and social sphere. It is an outcome of many conversations, dreams, disappointments and wishes of several years, converging on understanding the hidden psychological forces at play emerging from the functioning of the human psyche, especially in community settings – for individuals as well as for groups. All of us at Zeest have, through our own trajectories of working and engaging in the community-based social work, as well as through our practice in the clinic as psychoanalytically trained practitioners, come to appreciate the immense importance of understanding, reflecting on and engaging with the various psychological and unconscious underpinnings of our existence in a community and the cultural contexts. This understanding is needed before one begins to plan actions for creating impacts of various kinds at the social level. This is captured in the choice of the name of the organisation – 'Zeest', which means the very essence of existence. It also sounds like 'zeitgeist'.

As a part of the initial efforts, the organisation undertook to make an entry into engaging with psychoanalytic sensibilities to understand the experiences of people from the unorganised sector during the pandemic, as well as developing psychoanalytically informed methodology for engaging in socially relevant work. In this chapter we have compiled the experiences of people from the unorganised sector relating to the pandemic. Through semi-structured open-ended interviews, the researchers at Zeest tried to listen to the experiences of people working in this sector as they understood their own situation through the pandemic and how they made sense of the changes in their lives. Researchers at Zeest collaborated with MPhil students of psychoanalytic psychotherapy at Ambedkar University Delhi, who interned at Zeest for their community internship to conduct this study. The exercise was also undertaken to reflect on the process of entry into the community and making the initial contact for students of psychoanalysis. It was a part of an ongoing attempt to engage with social phenomena beyond their immediate impact and narration, rather as emotional situations and structures that actually shape our lived realities. It is important to listen to those whose voices have been drowned out by the sensationalistic buzz. More importantly, as psychoanalytic thinkers, it is important to listen to the 'unorganised' speech of those whose bodies can't resist speaking. The speech that bursts at the seams. The speech which is 'free' association and preserves the paradoxes, conflicts, interruptions, tentativeness, the slips, the negations and such undefined spontaneous presentations from the unconscious mind of the individual and the 'social' world dwelling inside the individual.

Making initial contact

A 65-year-old labourer, Yanis, works at a bakery in Mumbai. While recounting his experience of the pandemic, he repeated a few times, 'जब कोई सुनवाई नहीं है तो क्या कहें?' (*Jab koi sunvai nahi hai to kya kahein* – When there is no audience, no one to listen, what's the point of speaking?). He spoke with a sense of resignation. When asked about how he imagines recovery from the effects of the pandemic, he used the metaphor of someone having fallen into a ditch – 'गड्ढे में गिर गए तो निकलते निकलते ही निकलेंगे' (*gaddhe me gir gaye to nikalte nikalte hi niklenge* – when one has fallen in a ditch it will take time to come out to recover from the experiences of the pandemic). Yanis went back to his village after about a month and a half of the lockdown announcement. There were 20 people huddled in a cab. They met with police brutality at various points. There were children who were also facing hunger en route. He noted how the officials were most surprised when none of them tested positive for COVID-19 even though they were coming from a city which had a very high number of COVID patients at that time. At times they walked on foot. Their destination was in Uttar Pradesh (UP), over a thousand kilometres away.

Yanis just wishes for a new order. He has lost faith in any supportive structures. He mentioned fears and confusion about the pandemic. Personally, he wasn't sure what the big deal was about, yet he mentioned how at a time it was hard to find land for burials. He also reported fear of people being injected and killed. Yanis's no audience and so no speech struck sharply. A few times he also said, 'What can I say? I am a labourer.' Yanis was unemployed for over a year and a half and has just come back to Mumbai again to begin work. For the researcher, it felt like a door closing. Yanis seemed resigned and shut off. The metaphor of the ditch is at the cusp of a grave for which land is running out and a gradual ascending slope of a ditch from which emerging can be imagined. The 'not speaking' because no one will listen is also at this thin cusp. Is the complaint in the question – 'Why must I speak?' a flicker of hope emerging with the researcher's interest in listening to Yanis?

Zahir, another worker at a small bakery of buns in Mumbai, talked about a bitter experience of wanting to get back to his home in UP. When the lockdown was announced, all shops were shut. The money started running out.

They lived in a *chawl* (a community housing) and 15 men shared one room. Somehow, they arranged for food, but it was getting very tough for all of them in the room with no work. After a month and a half, they decided to go home anyway. They tried to escape in the back of a truck. They were found out. Police beat them up and sent them back. Later they decided to start the journey in auto rickshaws (three wheelers which are common public transport in urban India), four people in one auto rickshaw. They were again beaten up on the border. Some rickshaws' glass windshields were broken. They walked ahead, pulling the rickshaws on foot, and took a route through the countryside. People were leaving on foot, on bicycles. Zahir mentioned they carried a lot of water on them. On the way there were people begging to be carried in the rickshaw and on some vehicles. When they stopped to sleep, parking at a ghat, hordes of vehicles and trucks stopped behind to 'sleep'. All resting at night. When they reached UP, they were again beaten and slapped. There were some people offering food to the migrants along the way. When they reached their village people were being 'packed in plastics' and the villagers refused to speak to those arriving from other states. Zahir's description of foiled attempts to go back securely to his home in his village, to be with his family and to have some resources better than those in the city – available at the family home in terms of farmland and stored grains – made the researcher ask – 'Did you feel like crying?'. He replied:

> How can one cry in front of 15 people with whom you live! But we were all scared and feeling suffocated. There was a lot of anxiety. But we tried to encourage each other. We are young men! We even thought that we would go even if we got beaten or put in jail. It felt better to imagine being in jail, at least we would be given meals.

The fear of disease also was connected to being taken away to be killed. 'We were so scared to even cough. We would go to the bathroom if we had to cough or sneeze.' Zahir said one way that life is majorly affected going forward is that 'now no one helps monetarily anymore'. 'People don't borrow money and no one would help either.' He would even advise people to save for such adversities and not lend money to anyone. Zahir in his style of speaking inadvertently kept saying, 'समझ रहे हो?' (*Samajh rahe ho* – Are you getting it?). It sounded somewhere between 'can you understand' and 'it's not easy to understand'. Zahir is still a fairly well-to-do small-time businessman for buns and milk delivery. His narrative also brought in many people who were more unfortunate than him. Those begging to be given a lift on the way, a friend who had called to meet him but died of COVID (Zahir's friends told him he was lucky to have not met the friend otherwise he too would have contracted the disease) and a friend whose sister's wedding was called off due to financial losses of the family.

Akshay, a young musician, noted that there were significant differences in the way the world is around him now. When he used to perform earlier, a crowd would gather and pull him towards them, but now the audience he had was limited. He recalled that following one of the shows he did after the lockdown got lifted, he immediately came downstage and found for himself an isolated space as he did not want to come in contact with anyone. His quandary of coming into the audience and the crowd and now worrying about it and being isolated was an important one. It relates to our dilemma of entering into the community or remaining distanced from it. He shared that it was really disturbing to see the migrant workers going back home without any support from the government. He thought he should help them in some way. At the time, he along with a friend, collected 10,000 rupees and bought food, umbrellas, water pouches and chocolates to distribute to the people who were crossing the border which was near his house. When he reached the site, he saw a 'mob' of people coming towards him and they started asking him to give them money. It was really confusing for him as he could not understand what would they do with the money when everything is closed – they cannot buy tickets to go back and besides he was providing them food and water for their journey ahead. During the conversation the researcher sensed that he was angry at their demand for money. He thought to himself, 'why is money so important, everyone runs after money'. It almost felt like this greed that he perceived in the people for money had somehow made them less deserving of his compassion. He told them that he had no money. The researcher asked him, 'If you had known they would want money instead of the food and water, you would have given them money?' He said he would not have done so, because there is no limit to what amount of money you can offer to someone – it would not suffice. But if you offer someone food it satisfies a person for at least some time. Paradoxically, the musician also felt very cared for when his friend transferred money to his account during the lockdown. He mentioned later in the interview that he realised that money is also important after all! Something about money and its excess, an unsatisfiable want, is highlighted in Akshay's experience of being in the position of helper. Too much is being asked for; too much is being demanded. In his music, however, he resonates with this community's lack by trying to capture the anger and disappointment with the system which exacerbates these inequalities and injustices.

Another interview took place on the stairs of a construction site. Sunil, in his twenties, was from Bihar working far away from home in Karnataka. He felt supported and helped by the neighbouring grocery store which let him and his friends borrow rations. He brought up feeling helped in the community and appeared secure. The researcher asked him how he managed in the lockdown. His response surprised her. The labourer emphasised that he is able to make about a lakh in a year but it doesn't last because he needs to invest further and look after his family. He would have some savings to tide him over but not for such a long adversity. At the end, he thanked the researcher for 'someone big wanting to talk to someone small'. When the researcher asked what he meant by big, he said, 'elder, even if by a few months'. The researcher felt that Sunil was more secure financially than her. She was sitting below on the stairs, while Sunil was seated above during the interview. The interview seemed to challenge class division in a way. Sunil presented paradoxes about his situation. He also confounded the meaning of small and big as also experienced in the confusion of the researcher.

A vegetable seller who belonged to Bihar did not want to talk about the pandemic but felt the need to share his story of aspirations with the researcher. He shared with her that he had done masters and was teaching in Bihar but his college was not recognised and he couldn't get a government job. So, he came to Delhi in search of work and started selling vegetables. He wishes that his son will finish his education at a polytechnic and land a good job. He was happy to speak with the researcher bonding with her over her education. The fact that an educated young woman wanted to take his interview for 'research' made him relive his own intellectual dreams.

One of the interns shared her experience of working with another NGO which collaborated with the government to counsel people post-recovery. In one of her calls, she encountered a contractor who thought initially that she was a foreigner. It seemed he couldn't believe anyone would care in the country. When she clarified she was calling from Delhi, he first praised the government and then shared a list of complaints from his neighbourhood. When the researcher asked him to share his bodily condition and asked him to locate his pain, he said, 'There is pain in my heart'. The sea-saw of wanting and disbelief and disappointment in the contractor's narrative was interesting. He seemed disoriented about how much and what kind of help/concern would be apt from foreign lands versus closer home. That which was unimaginably 'distanced' seemed a more welcome and welcoming 'call', but that which felt like a closer contact invited more complaints and disappointments – 'a pain in the heart', at the core/centre of the concern.

Shobha, a housemaid who works in Delhi and whose family is in Bengal, shared her experience of being a single woman, having lost her alcoholic husband several years ago to an illness. She has two sons and a daughter, who are all married. Shobha brought up several times how she feels grateful that she was by herself. 'How could I have arranged food and stuff for more people?' Her son stayed with her initially in the lockdown as he had come to Delhi for some work. She was relieved when he could travel because the rations had started running out. She worried for her old mother who has respiratory issues and was back home in Bengal and felt she may never see her again. Towards the end of the interview, she wondered how difficult it could have been if her husband had been alive, since it would have been difficult to control him in his inebriated state. She talked about people who like getting intoxicated and don't care about others' safety, especially during the pandemic – those who don't wear masks and spit tobacco. Shobha preferred to be isolated but her mind went to all the people who could have caused chaos in her contained state. She could let her mind drift to those 'intoxicated' and uncontainable and spilling over, while securing her position by being at a distance from them in physical reality. Yet her mind was drifting to remember her dead alcoholic husband at this moment.

Anju, another housemaid, was scared, not knowing about the COVID disease when the pandemic started and feared she would be separated from her children. She also hoped that the interviewer wouldn't report anything to the police, for she feared that she would be taken away.

Irrational fears of being taken away by the police, being injected and killed for being sick, a lot of misinformation and paranoia were a part of most of the stories, apart from the nuanced paradox of 'distance' and 'contact'. It made us wonder if those not protected by any formal organisation felt the vulnerabilities of the pandemic to be persecutory and the government systems as wanting to get rid of them rather than help them. It captures the experience of feeling disenfranchised and being dispensable. At the same time, these paradoxes, confusions and hesitations only emerge with an offer to listen with no ask – freely speaking.

In conclusion

The various stories of not knowing what was happening to the world, to one's own body in the pandemic and the sudden shift in the social situation opened up many vulnerabilities based on uncertainties and insecurities.

One of the days as two researchers decided to walk along a road in Delhi to speak to some hawkers for these interviews, they noticed that a very familiar road near their residence was dotted with several small shanties and shops of a small nursery, a barber, a cobbler, a coconut water seller, some small tea stalls and so on. They had taken this route many times, yet during this pandemic situation when streets were fairly empty these small shops suddenly stood out. By virtue of being in the open space on the side of the road, they also brought up fears of contagion in the researchers as well. Before the pandemic it was easy to strike a conversation, sipping tea or getting a roadside haircut. Now making this contact seemed anything but casual and easy. It was easy to notice how their middle-class life was supported by so many service providers around in the community and yet reaching out and making contact had become so fraught. One had entered the phase of 'no-contact delivery'.

Another researcher, for her interview, visited a familiar market. She decided to talk to the street food vendor of *chaat* (spicy snack). She had been eating at his stall for several years. When she showed her interest to speak to this vendor, he agreed to meet her in the neighbourhood park to share his experiences. However, she was unable to meet him during this time. Later, when she visited his stall, she suddenly felt very conscious, as she felt he was staring at her chest. She started questioning her dress, while at the same time feeling very uncomfortable. We wondered in our reflective group if the 'stall guy' felt ashamed by the class difference between them and their vulnerabilities, and if this was his way of making her feel ashamed and cut off.

She had not experienced this discomfort earlier, so she decided to try again to close the interview, since this was in her neighbourhood and she was also concerned for her safety. This time again she felt very uncomfortable and too much stared at from behind. She also noticed that the man had a squint in his eyes. It was difficult for her to make sense of her experience while also taking into account this man's squint and his past behaviours before this encounter for the purpose of the interview.

Most of the researchers couldn't easily find participants for the interviews. It took days to set up the interview and decide the medium, and location to conduct the interview, not to mention to deal with the ambivalence of wanting to engage as well as wishing to maintain 'distance'.

Through these interviews, apart from listening to the stories of those whose lives we don't engage with, but on whose services we depend and who were affected very differently in the pandemic, we also discovered our own inhibitions, biases, vulnerabilities as well as difficulties of making a 'contact' which is taken for granted many times in social sciences and social work. We discovered that making the contact was by itself a psychoanalytic moment and a very important one to reflect on for social research and community work. It was worth noting through the experience of this research that an invitation for speaking freely, especially in the backdrop of lack of an individual voice and space, is also laboured with a 'pain in the heart'. It is important that the researcher bear the complaint in 'Why must I speak?' and 'Who will listen?'. These experiences during the pandemic of making contact and reaching into the community had acquired many different meanings. We only hope and wish that psychoanalysts and those interested in the in-betweens keep engaging with the struggle and speak and listen in the public domains to advocate for the free speech and freedom of speech to preserve our embodied subjectivity and recover it from falling into the ditch of fixed meanings and fixed locations and not make its grave in the landscape where there is no burial land left.

Acknowledgement

This chapter is an outcome of a research undertaken by Zeest: Centre for Psycho-Societal Innovation, Delhi, in collaboration with MPhil. Trainees of School of Human Studies, Ambedkar University Delhi. The researchers who have contributed to this work are Javed Ahmed, Khushboo Mehra, Shirine Marian Tigga and Varsha Jain

Notes

1 The meaning of a word is dynamic based on the context of its speech, its symbolic usage in a cultural context as well as in our unconscious mind where a word can only be a reference to some 'other' word. Freud highlighted this in his work on dream analysis. Words and images can be like metaphors and stand-ins for other

linking words and images by association. Lacan's work also highlights this aspect of our symbolic engagement with the world around us.

2 Transitional Space is a concept highlighted by Winnicott as the psychic space where the gap between 'me' and 'not me' and 'my productions' is not yet concretised. It's a creative space. It is also closer to Lacan's 'object a'.

3 In this work these metaphors drawn from actual experience during the pandemic are overlain and superimposed with a parallel boom of online (virtual) presence due to the need to maintain physical distance. This also seemed like a ripe opportunity for data-driven politics and business which extracts personal data for profit.

4 People working in non-formal, unincorporated, privately owned small enterprises or households. Many of these are daily wage earners and not on salaried income.

References

Beren, P., & Bach, S. (2018, June). Psychic space. *ROOM: A Sketchbook for Analytic Action.* https://analytic-room.com/essays/psychic-space/

Gentile, J. (2008). Between private and public: Towards a conception of the transitional subject. *The International Journal of Psychoanalysis, 89*(5), 959–976.

14 Unmasked

The dread of being able to kill

Urvashi Pawar

Introduction

Psychoanalytic work has survived the pandemic. The world as we know it has changed and we are all still reeling from the attack of this deadly coronavirus in our lives. It was in the early part of 2020 when patients started bringing in their fears of the virus. Before the lockdowns, when one was still meeting patients in person, one had not anticipated what lay ahead. There was probably a shared denial which sometimes still persists. It was in March of that year that the world shifted. In-person meetings turned to virtual ones and any space outside one's house was inaccessible. The air around us became toxic, human touch became deadly. The fears of contagion spread all around.

Suddenly, patients had to create the clinical setting in their own rooms and in their minds. From a three-dimensional world of the clinic, we shifted to a two-dimensional world of a computer screen. From a shared setting offered by the therapist, now there are two settings: the patient's room and the therapist's clinic.

Something other than the patient and the analyst and the co-created third had started entering the clinic. The virus, the fear of contagion and the dread of loss. Words feel meaningless at times and hope comes and goes.

A truth was emerging for all of us, we are all vulnerable and death can be just a breath away. One's sense of continuity and 'going-on-being' was under threat. Often one would experience it symbolically in the sessions when the network connectivity would fail. There was a shared panic, with the checking: 'Are you there?', 'Can you hear me/can you see me?' and I wondered whether it touched on our collective fears: Will we survive this?

Death and destructive drive

Only by the concurrent or mutually opposing action of the two primal instincts – Eros and the death-instinct – never by one or the other alone, can we explain the rich multiplicity of the phenomena of life.

(Freud, 1937, p. 243)

DOI: 10.4324/9781003255895-15

Psychoanalysis introduced the world to the idea that we humans harbour varied emotions and impulses. The human strives for health and growth and also within him has strivings which are aggressive and destructive in nature.

Freud (1937) elaborates on the ways the death drive manifests itself:

> If we take into consideration the total picture made up of phenomena of masochism immanent in so many people, the negative therapeutic reaction and the sense of guilt found in so many neurotics, we shall no longer be able to adhere to the belief that mental events are exclusively governed by the desire for pleasure. These phenomena are unmistakable indications of the presence of a power in mental life which we call the instinct of aggression or of destruction according to its aims, and which we trace back to the original death instinct of living matter.
>
> (p. 243)

Freud, in his 1920 paper 'Beyond the Pleasure Principle', introduced the idea of the death instinct and the duality of both the life instinct and the death instinct. He emphasized that an inclination to aggress and destroy is as fundamental to the human as the sexual instincts.

It was a Russian psychoanalyst Sabina Spielrein, one of the first few women psychoanalysts, who, in a paper written in 1912, 'Destruction as the Cause of Coming into Being', possibly paved the way for Freud's developing ideas on the death instinct.

> She talks about the different drives within the individual: The self-preservation drive is a 'static' drive, protecting the already existing individual against foreign influences. The drive for the preservation of the species is a 'dynamic' drive, which strives for transformation, the 'resurrection' of the individual in a new form. No transformation can proceed without the destruction of the old state.
>
> (Spielrein, 1912/1994, p. 174)

Freud's own ideas about death and destructive wishes started developing as he realised the need in the patients who had a 'Compulsion to Repeat' and often when working with patients who would not get better. He realised that there was more to the human psyche than the dualistic notion of Eros and sexual drives and the self-preservatory drives. His theories around the death drive developed along the years, and it culminated in one of his later works – 'Civilization and Its Discontents' (Freud, 1930). In it, he further elaborated how aggression was one of the primary derivatives of the death instinct.

Melanie Klein extended Freud's ideas of aggression and the death drive and helped us see how the struggle between love and hate, life and death, contribute to the psychic development of individuals. She was convinced about innate aggression in children and also developed her theoretical concepts through her clinical work with children. For Klein, annihilatory anxiety and the fear of fragmentation are experienced from very early on and form our primitive anxieties. These anxieties are defended against by very primary defence mechanisms, such as splitting, projection and introjection. In introducing the ideas of projection and projective identification, she helped us see how powerful and unformulated emotions from one's internal world can be placed outside and into another. These projections and projective identifications become important communications besides being defences to anxiety. Often death impulses are projected outwards and attach themselves onto primary external objects. There is a splitting that follows into good object and bad object. These objects furthermore can be introjected and become internal persecutors.

Though Klein focused on intrapsychic destructiveness, Wilfred Bion (1959) talked about how the destruction could be interpersonally and intrapsychically directed towards the relatedness and links to the object. Bion introduced us to the concept of the alpha function wherein beta elements (unprocessed and unformulated raw and minutely fragmented sense impressions) are converted to alpha elements (thinkable and visualizable elements). The alpha function is possible through the containing mind of a (m)other. Bion helped us see how destruction manifests in 'Attacks on linking' – when links between objects are destroyed because of the psychotic part of the personality. He introduces the idea of an ego-destructive superego where the ego itself is attacked from an internal object. In these attacks meaning-making and alpha function is destroyed.

Winnicott does not give much emphasis to the death instinct, and unlike Klein, he doesn't see destructiveness as an offshoot of the death instinct. He elaborates how the (m)other has to be created and destroyed in the child's fantasy. This also becomes a process of a transition from fantasy to reality. It is in the process of surviving the attack that the baby can see the mother as a real other who is not in one's omnipotent control. In talking about the unconscious fantasies that are a process of growth, Winnicott (1971/1989) says:

> If in the fantasy of early growth, there is contained death, then at adolescence there is contained murder. In the unconscious fantasy, growing up is inherently an aggressive act. . . . If the child is to become an adult, then this move is achieved over the dead body of the adult.
>
> (p. 144–145)

André Green brings in the notion of the Work of the Negative. Green (1999) explains how Thanatos could be working towards unbinding connections whereas the life instinct seeks to unite. In his view, one of the essential properties of the negative is to contest unity. He elaborates how the negative can be creative and structuring as much as it can be destructive.

Green (1999) developed the term 'disobjectalizing function' as the specific mode of action of the death drive in its opposition to the 'objectalizing function' of the life drives. According to him, the fundamental aim of the death drive is disinvestment and disengagement, and to destroy and withdraw from object relations. In these times when one is confronted and in grips with the workings of the negative, we see bereavement, loss and mourning, but we also see many people are creatively unshackling themselves from the everyday monotony of life.

Michael Eigen (1992) offers another vantage point, he says, 'One of the greatest weapons of the death drive is to make life appear to be unreal. One's sense of unreality may increase as the need to die in the face of one's owns sensitivity mounts' (p. 13).

Psychoanalysis aids the journey of tiding through all the emotions within and building the capacity to bear the unsufferable parts within us, to be able to suffer and heal. Our world of phantasies and dreams has room for hate and violence as much as it has place for love and compassion. There come times in history when one gets jolted out of the everyday turmoil into a situation where the world outside becomes too traumatic, and it brings alive buried and unprocessed parts of the internal world. Psychoanalysis approaches the understanding of our death and destructive instincts and its elaboration in our development from various perspectives. A multiple-vertices approach becomes useful in understanding difficult emotions. Given the present environment, it becomes important to develop a nuanced listening to the workings of these internal forces and how they are re-evoked.

The caesura of COVID

It was an ordinary day in January 2020, when the news of coronavirus, or then called Wuhan Virus, started creating a stir. It was initially othered, kept far away. No one had imagined how it would sweep in and storm into every individual's body and mind. Life as we know it has changed. There is a caesura that has now been created.

Bion (1967, 1977/1989) developed the idea of a caesura, taking from Freud's words about the 'Impressive Caesura of birth'. Caesura indicates a break and continuity; how does one make meaning of this time? Bion reminded us to investigate the caesura. We together are building a capacity within to observe the caesura of COVID.

If we think of the caesura of birth, the new-born enters the world and has to lose the womb in the process of coming into the world. In that very moment so much changes. Separations are inevitable, as life progresses many such endings are necessary so as to move to another experience. Where the old is, the new shall be. One sees what was and goes on to create the space for the new.

The dread of the virus became an important truth in all the sessions with our patients. One week we were in the room with our patients in flesh and blood, and the next week suddenly we became two-dimensional screens or a voice in the ear. The therapy space has been attacked; the sensorial experience has been taken away. Usually when there is a break in therapy or the setting or even timings of sessions, it evokes a strong wave of emotions. Change brings with it a storm of emotions and associations. The internal and psychical rhythms change. When the virus started spreading and lockdown was declared without much preparation, suddenly there was a rupture. A loss which couldn't be grieved. There wasn't a place for anger or blame. Patients and therapists accepted this change and it was a strange separation with no definite certainty. It is hard to say where the other side of the pandemic lies, it is hard to say with certainty when would it be safe to meet each other. But there is continuity, life is moving.

Bergstein (2013) says:

> The psychoanalytic quest is not traversing the caesura so as to arrive at a safe harbor, but rather widening the capacity for motion and free flowing between the two river banks, between the two rims of the caesura. The mere movement and transition are what matters and not its *direction*, hence there is no notion of moving forward towards a goal, or cure. *The movement itself* is what expands the mind and facilitates psychic life.
>
> (p. 625)

So in some ways, we were all striving for movements, and paradoxically there is a search for stillness while bearing a force from outside. The sense of the caesura helps us to traverse these times. Even though there is a shared truth of the pandemic, it is a unique caesura for every person.

Confronting the dread of causing the illness: What emerges in the clinic

The reality of the contagion doesn't allow us to meet in person. Our bodies are not safe spaces; one can infect the other unknowingly. At one level there are persecutory and annihilatory anxieties and at another there is a fear of losing a loved one. At a level deeper lies our oedipal anxieties, our murderous phantasies and fears of punishment and guilt.

The question often comes up, who caused a loved one to get it? One can't help blame themselves, homicidal accusations haunt everyone. Often one denies this responsibility and places it anywhere but on themselves. While many grieve and mourn, those who have lost a loved one are haunted by the truth of how the virus insidiously took the life of their family member or friend. In our society when isolation and lockdowns has meant living together with family, each family member carries a shared responsibility and guilt of wondering whether they could cause the illness. It affects everyone, plagues those families who have suffered a loss and those who have escaped it.

Freud (1912) writes about the death of a loved one:

> [T]he survivor is overwhelmed by tormenting doubts (to which we give the name of 'obsessive self-reproaches') as to whether she may not herself

have been responsible for the death of this cherished being through some act of carelessness or neglect. . .. We find that in a certain sense these obsessive self-reproaches are justified, and this is why they are proof against contradictions and protests. It is not that the mourner was really responsible for the death or was really guilty of neglect, as the self-reproaches declare to be the case. Nonetheless, there was something in her-a wish that was unconscious to herself- which would not have been dissatisfied by the occurrence of death and which might actually have brought it about if it had had the power. And after death *has* occurred, it is against this unconscious wish that the reproaches are a reaction.

(p. 60)

The therapist listens to what has been silenced in our patients but might be terrorizing screams from within. The patients might deny their destructive wishes and also then deny the external truth of the destructive powers of the virus. Many people might become more risky and not cautious either as a self-destructive or an aggressive act. Some might become very afraid of the virus and fear the attack or punishment of their aggressive wishes. People get immersed in guilt, often persecutory in nature. Persecutory anxieties heighten, fearing that all the aggression that one had placed outside could come to attack back.

In psychoanalysis, patients confront ambivalent feelings towards their parents, siblings, lovers and friends. Freud (1912) says:

In almost every case where there is an intense emotional attachment to a, we find that behind the tender love there is a concealed hostility in the unconscious. This is the classic example, the prototype, of the ambivalence of human emotions.

(p. 60)

Similarly, Eigen suggests, 'The deepest bonds call forth the most aggression, at the same time the latter is incessantly displaced. A perennial problem with aggression is that wherever it goes, it boomerangs. No movement is final' (2001, p. 138). During the pandemic, it has become harder to express hostile feelings. Patients are bringing in their fears, the fear of death, their imagination about getting ill and the toxic spread of the virus. They fear becoming carriers; the unknowability of it all is scary.

In these uncertain times, the continuity of sessions possibly made the fragilities of this time more bearable. The dread of loss through this time is a shared truth. Aggressive phantasies and violent emotions become harder to express. It feels too overwhelming. The boundary between reality and phantasy seems too thin. Often elaborations of enraged and angry feelings towards others and also towards the therapist stopped emerging in the sessions. For some patients, getting therapy and having a therapist to care for them evoked guilt.

It becomes important to establish that though the porosity of our bodies make us vulnerable and susceptible to the virus, it is through the porosity of our mind that we seek strengthening. The therapist's mind is a porous container that offers itself to the other. This terror emerges in the dyad often in disguised ways, in the transference and countertransference, in enactments. The patient's fears will be felt by the therapist if the patient is able to feel less afraid of burdening or contaminating the therapist's capacity to metabolize. Laplanche and Pontalis (1973) write that in Freud's final instinctual theory 'aggressiveness must certainly be seen as a radical force for disorganization and fragmentation' (p. 21).

The work of analysis then entails offering the patient a mind which can create an organizing function and a place where the fragmented parts can be deposited safely and where emotional experiences can seek comprehension. But this process has also been hard for some patients in these times as there is a concern about the well-being of the therapist as well. When the survivability of the analyst is in question, patients become unable to express their anger and vulnerability easily. Regardless of the pre-condition that Winnicott helped us prepare for as practitioners 'The Analyst Survives' – in these present times it is under threat. It becomes important to not evade this reality but also to be able to show that at the moment you both are alive.

Movements within and moments of transformations: Building psychic antibodies and bearing the uncertainty

We shall take years to recognize how the world has changed because of the pandemic. One would argue that these terrors are a continuation of the terrors that haunt us from childhood, terrors that have been successfully and unsuccessfully repressed (or probably were too primal to have been repressed). It's a different kind of Unknown. It can't be equated and it is unfamiliar.

I say this because there is another layer present in this dread. It's the dread of a real death and a death that can be given to another without any act of violence but because of a spread of a virus. Meltzer (1986) says that one of the fundamental benefits of analysis is a movement from a causal/explanatory attitude, which attributes guilt, to an attitude that seeks to understand and accept the uncertainty that is inherent in the infinite complexity of the human development and personal relations.

What is emerging are unmentalized emotional experiences. Meaning-making in these times is not easy and as analysts we might not have always been able to contain, hold and process. In these times what has mattered is that the analyst intends to make meaning and offer themselves to the patients' terrors and grief while also holding the dread of the external reality for them and bearing the reverberance of the past and the fears of the present. What matters is an authentic at-one-ment (Bion) with each other.

Bion, taking from the poet John Keats offered the idea of 'negative capability' as 'capable of being in uncertainties, mysteries, doubts, without any

irritable reaching after fact and reason' (Bion, 1970, p. 125). In these traumatic times, primitive fears seem like 'beta – elements' almost like the virus
in the air seeking a body to inhabit. The therapist's mind and body can offer
a space which doesn't become contagious and work towards turning the
beta elements to alpha elements. This also includes creating a capacity to
bear the to and fro of the process.

If we were to consider the metaphor of cure in the terminology of the
COVID-19 virus, we can see that what appears to offer protection is the
creation of antibodies. The body's immune system is activated when one is
infected or vaccinated and an internal war ensues between the attacking
virus and the defending antibodies. Often one is facing a similar psychological war when one is struggling emotionally. We are trying to create psychic
antibodies – the process of destruction in order for preservation. We seek
the destructive function also as a way to protect and create. When humans
defend, they also destroy.

There can be times in a human's life when this destructive force is not
reined in and can overwhelm the person. At these times, the threat of overwhelming rage and violence threaten psychic equilibrium. Primitive defence
mechanisms provide temporary solace. When the rage is placed outside
and projected, often the external objects become threatening, and when it's
introjected, internal attacks ensue.

We confront the handicap of language and experiences that cannot be
put into words. When very primitive, unrepresented and ineffable emotions
emerge in the virtual clinic the therapist can often contain them, often have
dreams or nightmares with and for her patients and in the course of the
sessions the reveries and countertransference experiences become available guiding forces. Often therapists also touch raw and unprocessed parts
within their psyche. They touch on their fears of loss and death and their
own aggressive and terrorizing parts. Ogden (2005) talks about the analyst
partaking in dreaming the patient's undreamt and interrupted dreams. In
these unbearable times, there is a caesura that has been created in people's
capacity to dream and to free-associate. The work of the therapist is to traverse the undreamt nightmares and even more overwhelming reality for their
patients and for themselves as well.

César and Sára Botella (2015) offer a direction which is useful at these times
where the journey involves moving from unrepresentable states towards representation. They suggest that this process of intelligibility and 'figurability'
requires the analyst to regress in the course of the sessions along with the
patient but come out from that state of possibly unthinkable horror to a state
of being able to find a representation and create symbolic meaning and then
offer it to the patient. This regression means the analyst getting in touch with
her own internal conflicts, primitive anxieties, and being able to recover from
it, and through this contagious experience, in the session with the patient,
also show the parts which survive the contagion. This sort of immersion
which is experienced allows a felt experience of the patient's world.

In the end we endeavour to mourn the loss of the past and the recent loss of the present and recover and repair the psyche of that which shall always be missing. In these times, therapy involves creating a space to mourn, grieve and also preserve and protect the inherent aggressive and creative aspects of our psyche. Our work then entails unmasking this dread of being able to kill. I conclude with Hanna Segal's (1952) words:

> [A]ll creation is really a re-creation of a once loved and once whole, but now lost and ruined object, a ruined internal world and self. It is when the world within us is destroyed, when it is dead and loveless, when our loved ones are in fragments, and we ourselves in helpless despair – it is then that we must re-create our world anew, re-assemble the pieces, infuse life into dead fragments, re-create life.
>
> (p. 199)

References

Bergstein, A. (2013). Transcending the caesura: Reverie, dreaming and counter-dreaming. *International Journal of Psychoanalysis, 94,* 621–644.

Bion, W. R. (1959). Attacks on linking. *International Journal of Psycho-Analysis, 40,* 308–315.

Bion, W. R. (1967). A theory of thinking. In *Second thoughts: Selected papers on psychoanalysis.* Heinemann.

Bion, W. R. (1970). *Attention and interpretation.* Tavistock Publications.

Bion, W. R. (1989). *Two papers: 'The grid' and 'Caesura'.* Karnac Books. (Original work published 1977)

Botella, C., & Botella, S. (2015). *The work of psychic figurability: Mental states without representation* (A Weller with the collaboration of M Zerbib, Trans.). Brunner-Routledge.

Eigen, M. (1992). *Coming through the whirlwind: Case studies in psychotherapy.* Chiron Publications.

Eigen, M. (2001). *Damaged bonds.* Routledge.

Freud, S. (1912–1913). Totem and taboo. In J. Strachey (Ed.), *The standard edition of the complete psychological works of Sigmund Freud, Vol. 13.* Hogarth Press.

Freud, S. (1920). Beyond the pleasure principle. In J. Strachey (Ed.), *The standard edition of the complete psychological works of Sigmund Freud, Vol. 18.* Hogarth Press.

Freud, S. (1930). Civilisation and its discontents. In J. Strachey (Ed.), *The standard edition of the complete psychological works of Sigmund Freud, Vol. 21* (pp. 57–145). Hogarth Press.

Freud, S. (1937). Analysis terminable and interminable. In J. Strachey (Ed.), *The standard edition of the complete psychological works of Sigmund Freud, Vol. 23* (pp. 209–254). Hogarth Press.

Green, A. (1999). *The work of the negative* (A. Weller, Trans.). Free Association Books.

Laplanche, J., & Pontalis, J. B. (1973). *The language of psycho-snalysis* (D. Nicholson-Smith, Trans., The International Psycho-Analytical Library, Vol. 94, pp. 1–497). The Hogarth Press and the Institute of Psycho-Analysis.

Meltzer, D. (1986). *Studies in extended metapsychology: Clinical applications of Bion's ideas.* Clunie Press.

Ogden, T. H. (2005). *This art of psychoanalysis: Dreaming undreamt dreams and interrupted cries.* Routledge.

Segal, H. (1952). A psycho-analytical approach to aesthetics. *The International Journal of Psychoanalysis, 33*, 196–207.

Spielrein, S. (1994). Destruction as the cause of coming into being. *Journal of Analytical Psychology, 39*(2), 155–186. (Original work published 1912)

Winnicott, D. W. (1989). *Playing and reality.* Routledge. (Original work published 1971)

15 Where are your brains?

Anurag Mishra, Bhaskar Mukherjee and Anup Dhar

Introduction: Doctors (past and present) in dialogue

Focusing on the problem of 'brain', the following tripartite dialogue between Anurag Mishra, Bhaskar Mukherjee and Anup Dhar is the result of Livonics's effort to explore how contemporary interdisciplinary thinking can challenge *preconceptions* about body, mind and their relations, as also about psychotherapy and psychoanalysis. The trialogue – which happens between the second and the third wave – examines in both a 'disruptive and integrative' manner the intertwined foldings of the neuronal, the linguistic and the affective bodies. The Livonics Institute of Integrated Learning and Research (LIILR) was born between the first and the second wave of the COVID-19 pandemic. It was itself a response to the pandemic. It was a response to the new questions we were facing in the larger sphere of 'mental health' during the pandemic, including what lockdown, quarantine and social distancing could do to human species. Questions pertaining to how vulnerable the human is faced with the madness of the tiniest organism, the virus, looked pertinent. Questions pertaining to how one needed to think anew at the interface of the natural and the human sciences and not restrict oneself to either the natural or human science silos seemed urgent. For LIILR the question is not whether psychotherapy or psychoanalysis will be or can be conducted online; important as it is, it is a question of just the 'setting'. The more important question is: how do we make sense of the human and the non-human brain-mind complex in the twenty-first century; what kind of new philosophical, scientific and socio-cultural question is the pandemic throwing up? This trialogue is an effort in that direction, not to clinch one position in favour of the other, not to pit one position against the other, but to dialogue with patience and with care.

Dr Anurag Mishra: Good morning. I am the founder of the Livonics Institute of Integrated Learning and Research (LIILR), where we focus on disruptive and integrated learning and research. I am fond of quoting my favourite philosopher Alan Watts, who once famously said

DOI: 10.4324/9781003255895-16

that 'problems that remain persistently insoluble should always be suspected as questions asked in the wrong way'. We at Livonics focus on asking questions and finding answers through the simultaneous use of multiple lenses, underpinned by the belief that we can see clearly with the addition of different disciplinary lenses to the pre-existing ones, much like by going to an optometrist we can see the writing on the wall in a clearer way. Today we are going to be doing something quite disruptive, maybe even explosive. However, first I will talk about this question which is the topic of our conversation; and I think 'conversation' is a very civilised way to deal with questions rather than lectures or other things like that. So, the story of this topic began more than 30 years ago, when I was in school and was supposed to be attending a lecture on *Macbeth* I suspect. But I was looking out of the window at a rather attractive lady. Which my teacher noticed and then asked me with some irritation, 'Where are your brains?' This is a question which I have been trying to answer for a very long time, and in this long time my fickle brain has gone from engineering to medicine to psychiatry to psychoanalysis and then to a host of other disciplines. Which made many people, including me, wonder whether I had at least lost my mind if not my brain! During this somewhat nomadic phase of my life which I will try to illustrate, I met like-minded nomads and gypsies of the mind, two of whom are my panellists today. And I must say that everybody in Livonics is absolutely peripatetic, nobody is ever to be found in the same place twice. This is a very important point because all of them have travelled intellectually to many disciplines. For example, Dr Bhaskar Mukherjee has travelled from psychiatry to neuroscience to molecular medicine and then to neurogenetics. Professor Anup Dhar was a medical professional and a left political activist who through post-structural critiques of mental health arrived at a rethought form of psychoanalysis and through postcolonial critiques of the Left arrived at a rethought form of the political. Both of them are now senior fellows at LIILR, and along with them we have at Livonics many other nomads and gypsies of mind, body and soul as our audience today. I welcome you all. I welcome Dr Bhaskar Mukherjee, who calls himself a student of psychiatry. He loves to understand and evaluate the pathophysiological basis of psychiatric symptoms, both macro- and microscopically. His journey from connectomics to genomics is motivated by his interests in areas like treatment resistance in and trans-diagnostics understanding of psychiatry. His life's goal is to make psychiatry regain the master spot in medicine – a spot reserved for 'speciality' in medicine dealing with the master organ of the body. So Bhaskar, tell us what is our brain? Where is it? And, why is it one of the most important organs?

The master organ

Dr Bhaskar Mukherjee: From my perspective, I would not say *it* (the brain) is 'one of the most important' but rather I would always say that the brain is the *most important* organ. In fact, I would request all of you to close your eyes and imagine an organism which consists of a brain, two protruding eyeballs and a tail-like spinal cord, all connected through a group of nerves hanging down the body. If you can visualise this organism. This organism is actually 'us'. The rest of the body is just an exo-suit that the organism wears. The foremost question any one of you could raise at this moment would be that *Is the rest of the body not us?* And I would say, *Not us* because if we follow the advances in transplantation sciences, we know that everything other than 'this organism' is replaceable, be it our limbs, heart, kidneys, skin or muscles. Only this organism that I talked about previously cannot be replaced. Our brain, spinal cord and eyes cannot be transplanted. These are the parts that make us human beings. If we remove or change any of these areas, the organism changes.

The brain is the master organ of this whole exoskeleton. It controls this exoskeleton and every organ of the body through many layers: the first and second layers that are physical in nature are the immune and neuro-endocrine systems, through various hormones and intricate neural connections. There is no organ in our body that does not receive direct signals from the brain. Initially, it was thought that the bone marrow does not contain neural connections but recently it has come to our knowledge that bone marrow, lymph nodes, all of them have their own neural connections that help them in carrying out their life cycles. The third layer is *reality*. When we see reality, we have to understand that we are not seeing anything real but rather we are seeing an artificial overlay of reality created by our brain. Starting from the day one of postnatal life, it creates our reality. Let us say, I am seeing someone playing on a football field. And I do not have a special attraction for football. So, for me my reality would be that someone is playing in a field with a football and some other people are seeing that. And I would associate that with my fear of too many people or my personal dislike for organised social structure and other things and I would create a reality of my own. Now replace me with some other brain which loves and follows cricket and finds everything associated with cricket very exciting. Now that person would see this football game very differently and that brain would create its own meaning. Now if we take another brain, that of a football enthusiast, it would be overjoyed by the sight of that football game and would create another reality. I have just given a single example of a game to show the associated feelings and three different realities created by three different brains. Now take everything in our environment that we see has for us a 'memory-engram': which is a part of our memory that we have learnt previously and have some special meaning of that thing in our brain. And you would now understand that there can be 'n' number of realities that can be created out of social stimuli by our brains. In that sense, the brain becomes the most important organ of ours.

Then comes the external environment which we call 'society'; that is also created by our brains. For this we have to understand that humans are 'hive' organisms such that every cell in our body has its own life cycle, and the brain is the combined result of those interdependent and interactive life cycles. Now take each individual as that single cell having a life cycle. In that sense, our society is a *hive-organism* where each of these brains interact and form a complex megastructure of a mega-animal. Why has humanity become the *apex* predator of our ecosystem? We do not have anything special like sharp teeth or claws; or special physical powers like other animals, as we are neither good swimmers or runners nor can we fly. We are not good at anything. But yet today, 20 million years after the human species originated, human beings are the apex predators of this ecosystem. However, if we take a single member of the human species and put him/her in a wilderness, they would die and be killed by various other animals. Because singularly human beings would fare somewhere at the bottom to middle of the ecological pyramid. But if you join a group of humans and create a society, then that society would become a mega-animal and would then dominate every other animal on the ecological pyramid. And that 'joining' of individuals into a society is again an attribute of the brain. It starts at a very primitive mammalian level. If you think about whales, they have a primitive society. Even in the case of non-mammalians like ants, they have a primitive society. But as human brains are considered as more developed in various aspects, it has structured understandings of how to join other brains through various means such that of (verbal) communication, knowledge sharing and so on. In that sense, human society due to the human brain(s) is truly a multi-appended single organ. And that organ is the master of Earth's ecological pyramid. So if we now ask again, 'Where is our brain?', then we can say that the brain is *the organ that we are*; and which communicates with other such organs and by conjoining creates a society, which is a higher-level organism or animal that now rules over this planet called Earth and its ecosystem. It is ruling very badly, no doubt, but it is ruling nonetheless. So in a very schematic view, this is where our brains are – everywhere and also inside our skulls.

Dr Anurag Mishra: This is good and bad. Good because Bhaskar you have said more or less what I was planning to say and I thought I would be the first one to say it! So, it is good that we are both on the same page. And bad because now I am going to run short of things to say eventually. But humour aside, somebody asked me about this conversation, this dialogue – to whom is it addressed? And who is going to understand all of it? To which I said nobody is going to understand all of it. Because somebody will understand something or the other according to their respective positions and interests. And a small section of people for whom I think this is going to be important are those who do not know everything. As for the people who know everything, neither this nor any of the courses at Livonics are of any use. This is for people who are really interested in the mysteries of the world and want to understand and are willing to travel from one place to another; only they would appreciate what we are talking about. Professor Anup Dhar, would you please shed more light on this question?

The question of consciousness

> . . . *there is, within each human being, no [One] Brain, only some brains.*
> (Alan Badiou)

Dr Anup Dhar: Building on the metaphor of *driving*, which requires an integration of *windscreen* and *rear-view* images and perspectives, this short response to the question 'where is your brain' shall argue for the need to bring to dialogue the following:

1   Rear-view perspectives in psychoanalysis (where we get to see 'early Freud' – Freud the neurobiologist and not just the metapsychological Freud; we see the *origins* of psychoanalysis; we see *originary multiplicity* at the origin of psychoanalysis; we see *ab-Original* insights – insights that put into question the 'original insights').
2   The windscreen views (we see contemporary advances in neurobiology – affective neuroscience – in this view as also contemporary advances in philosophy – especially neurophilosophy).

It shall also argue for bringing to dialogue (1) *natural science* and (2) *human science* (one can take a look at the edited volume *Breaking the Silo* for such a dialogue in the Indian context) insights on what Jaak Panksepp calls the integrated Brain-Mind system (I would like to designate it as the *Mind-Brain Moebius*).

One of the questions this conversation has to contend with is the question of 'consciousness'. The framework that has dominated our understanding of consciousness is that consciousness could be reduced to physical and chemical elements. Freud also tried to develop a 'natural science of the mind' so as to explore the 'quantitatively determinate states of specifiable material particles' in the *Project* (1895/1953). He failed in his project, lacking the tools and methods (thinkers are limited by the tools of their times – both conceptual and technological), and abandoned it to move to metapsychology; the *Aphasia* book signalled the turnaround. This turn to metapsychology gave birth to psychoanalysis but also severed the connection psychoanalysis could have had with natural science questions.

Coming back to the question of consciousness, David Chalmers (1996) showed that the search for the neural correlates of consciousness was an 'easy' problem. It was a correlational solution rather than a causal one. The neural correlates could tell us something about the 'where' of the origin of consciousness; it doesn't tell us much about *'why' and 'how' consciousness arises* (the same can be said about the unconscious; Freud stretches himself to the limit to make sense of the why and how of the unconscious in 'The Unconscious' paper [1915/1957]). For Chalmers, the 'hard' problem of consciousness was: how and why do neurophysiological activities produce the experience of consciousness (or of *intentionality*)? Why don't we see the world like a camera? How do we make sense of the experience of *see-ing*? The hard problem, therefore, is: why and how does the subjective quality of experience arise from objective neurophysiological events?

Contrary to popular belief, Mark Solms shows how 'objectivity and subjectivity are observational perspectives', not 'cause and effect'. Neuronal locations (the *where* [in the brain] question) are *not* the cause of consciousness; they are mere correlations (nor can they be the cause of the unconscious); just like lightning is not the cause of thunder; they are correlates; they are parallel manifestations of a third process: *electricity*. The *why* and *how* of consciousness studies shall perhaps be a search for that *elusive third* in the coming years.

We usually describe the underlying causes of biological phenomena in 'functional' terms, and functional mechanisms can in turn be reduced to natural laws. For example: what is the mechanism of vision? However, Chalmers correctly points out that the functional mechanism of vision does not explain *what it is like to see* or *what it is like to be a bat* a la Thomas Nagel. This is because vision is not an intrinsically conscious function. The performance of visual functions (even specifically human ones, like read-*ing*) need not have the *feel of seeing*; microscopes and telescopes 'see' – perhaps far better and far more than humans – without the experience or feel of see-*ing*. Perception can occur without an awareness of what is perceived. Therefore, Chalmers reasonably asked: 'Why is the performance of these functions accompanied by experience? Why doesn't all this information processing go on 'in the dark', free of any inner feel?' How do we make sense of what Merleau-Ponty calls *intentionality*? Wittgenstein in *Philosophical Investigations* suggests: 'only of a human being and what resembles (behaves like) a living human being can one say: it has sensations; it sees, is blind; hears, is deaf; is conscious or unconscious'.

Chalmers's question may reasonably be asked of all cognitive functions, not only visual ones, but the same does not apply to affective functions. How can you have a feeling without feeling it? How can we explain the functional mechanism of affect without explaining why and how it causes us to experience something? Even Freud agreed on this score: 'It is surely of the essence of an emotion that we should be aware of it, i.e. that it should become known to consciousness.'

What is it like to look at one's body in the mirror? It looks to be an entity extended in space; it looks objectifiable, at least, up to an extent; it looks like a kind of materiality. What is it to close one's eyes thereafter? Does one have a feel of one's own body? One has, perhaps. One could call such a 'feel' the lingering image of one's past vision of one's body in the mirror. But then, we have similar feelings for the body even in dreams, as also even if one is blind. It appears they are the same body; there is, however, no substance dualism, but there is a dualism of perspective; are they two different means of comprehending one and the same reality? Hence the need to think along a Mind-Brain Moebius. Further, how do we engage with both in their mutual constitutivity: their overdetermination; how do we integrate both views: causally? Or functionally? How does one work through what Marx calls *mechanical materialism* (body-to-mind causality) and *mind-body dualism*? How does one negotiate between transcendental idealism and mechanical materialism? How does one connect the *in vitro* and the *in vivo*? How does one work through objective/subjective, third person/first person accounts? Further, how does one engage then with the person? The person (even if barred as subject)?

Building on the 'hard' problem of consciousness: the causal *how* and *why* do neurophysiological activities produce the experience of consciousness (and not just the correlational *where*), I would like to ask: is consciousness exclusively cortical? Is it just a cognitive function? Or is consciousness an affective function as well; which is only secondarily 'extended' upwards to the 'higher' perceptual and cognitive mechanisms that Freud described as the systems Pcpt.-Cs. and Pcs (as Solms and Panksepp argue)? Does the corticocentric view of the human not let us see how the 'higher' functions might depend on the integrity of its 'lower' structures? Do we then need to rethink the relationship between 'higher' and 'lower' in the sciences? Did the philosophical distinction between mind and body come to coincide with the anatomical distinction between the cortex and the phylogenetically 'ancient' subcortex? What then could be the dialectic between internal states of the (visceral, autonomic) body and external perceptions; between *autoaffection* and *apperception*, *inner* and *outer* (and not just higher and lower)? Would this also lead to a reconsideration of the relationship between language/ signifier and affect in psychoanalysis?

Through the nineteenth century the cortex had become the organ of the mind and the subcortical brain had become mindless. The peripheral sensory-motor parts and the innate and subcortical parts, including the parts that transmit impressions from the inside of the body, were considered to be purely reflex. Thus, the philosophical distinction between mind and body had come to coincide with the anatomical distinction between the cortex and the subcortex.

In this context, it is of utmost importance to work our way through the top-down *corticocentric* view of the Mind-Brain Moebius (including perhaps an over-privileging of grey matter) and the subsequent designation of certain areas as *sub*cortical, as lower, as inferior. Contemporary advances in affective neuroscience argue for an *affective consciousness from below*, from what has been incorrectly designated '*sub*cortical areas'. Cortical functioning looks to be accompanied by consciousness only if it is 'enabled' by the reticular activating system of the upper brainstem. Solms and Panksepp (2012) show how damage to just two cubic millimetres of this region obliterates consciousness. The consciousness generated by the upper brainstem also has *qualitative content* of its own. This could be designated *affect* – affect as the in-between thought and action. Since cortical consciousness is contingent upon brainstem consciousness, affect is revealed to be the foundational form of consciousness. The sentient subject is literally constituted by affect. In this view, as Mark Solms suggests: 'Since the cerebral cortex is the seat of intelligence, almost everybody thinks that it is also the seat of consciousness. . .. Consciousness is far more primitive than that. It arises from a part of the brain that humans share with fishes'. This is the 'hidden spring' of affective consciousness. Perception itself is a nonconscious process, and begs the question: what does consciousness add to perception? The answer from Solms and Panksepp: *consciousness adds feeling*.

The cerebral sites that produce emotion occupy a zone which starts at the level of the brain stem and goes up to the cortex. Outside of a part of the frontal lobe called the prefrontal ventromedial cortex, the majority of these sites are 'subcortical'. The principal subcortical sites are located in regions of the brain stem, the hypothalamus and the basal telencephalon. The amygdala is a determinant subcortical site in the triggering of emotions. The upper brainstem structures that generate consciousness do not map our external senses; they map the internal state of the (visceral, autonomic) body.

Josef Parvizi (2009) argues in a paper titled 'Corticocentric Myopia: Old Bias in New Cognitive Sciences' how 'the cerebral cortex is seen to have the most important role in 'higher' functions of the brain, such as cognition and behavioral regulation, whereas subcortical structures are considered to have subservient or no roles in these functions'. Parvizi highlights 'the conceptual bias at the root of this corticocentric view of the human brain'; he in the process 'emphasizes its negative implications in current practices in the cognitive neurosciences'. The corticocentric view of the human brain is also a myopic view because it does not let us see that the purportedly higher functions depend on the integrity of the 'phylogenetically ancient subcortical structures, and by the instinctual and affective processes associated with themits lower structures'.

Further, as Damasio, Farah, Huerta and Ramachandran suggest in the *Encyclopedia of the Human Brain*,

> no single psychological concept fully describes the functions of any given brain area or circuit. There are no unambiguous 'centres' or loci

for discrete emotions in the brain that do not massively interdigitate with other functions, even though certain key circuits are essential for certain emotions to be elaborated. Everything ultimately emerges from the interaction of many systems.

For this reason, contemporary neuroscientists talk about interacting 'circuits', 'networks', and 'cell assemblies' rather than 'centres'. This would entail a movement from the earlier 'centres' to *overdetermined assemblages of complex configurations*.

Let me end with a statement on the course titled 'Psychoanalysis in Practice: Between Philosophy and Neuroscience', which LIILR is about to launch. This course is not born out of *knowingness*. It is born out of doubt; self-doubt; doubts that poetically fold back upon us, upon our certainties, our rigidities. What might psychoanalytic practice look like if sincere and sustained efforts are made to integrate the many implications flowing from cutting-edge neuroscience research? We begin by delineating the limits of psychoanalytic practice when it is faced with revelations arising from new scientific investigations of the brain; ignoring the advances of neurobiology perhaps lands the 'theorist of subjectivity' in metaphysical dogmatism. It will thereafter ask: can psychoanalysis and neuroscience mutually enrich each other if brought to dialogue and integrated with care; is philosophy the missing link between the two? Both the psychoanalytic and neuroscientific sides of this 'hybrid interdisciplinary formation' (with streaks of integration and interruption) may have to be dialectically rethought: one perhaps needs neuroscientific psychoanalysis and a psychoanalytic neuroscience. Neither psychoanalysis nor the neurosciences (nor philosophy) can remain unchanged in passing through these unavoidable disciplinary intersections, and negotiating between apparently incommensurable disciplinary regimes, like philosophy and neurobiology, and historically separated knowledge registers, like the human and the natural sciences. Would such a *negotiation* birth a new understanding of the unconscious as *structured like an uncanny homeostasis*?

> **Dr Anurag Mishra:** Anup, this question that you have raised about mind-body (you call it the Mind-Brain Moebius) as also about inside-outside and their relationship is akin to the kind of question Winnicott raised while talking about transitional objects – a question that should not be asked to the child. In his words:
>
>> It is a matter of agreement between us and the baby that we will never ask the question whether you conceived of this or was it presented to you from without. The important point is that no decision on this is to be expected, the question is not to be formulated.
>
> So questions like what is inside and what is outside, what is brain and mind, rather are two aspects of the same coin or are in a *Moebius relationship* if one were to look at it that way. As I was looking at

that attractive lady, my mind was distracted by her, or I may even be said to have lost my mind, which actually also means that we have lost our heart! But in all these, what of the brain? The heart is the realm of poets, artists and single malt whiskeys. And the mind is the realm of serious psychoanalysts, who usually do not say many things and rock on their chairs and do frequent 'hmms' and 'huhs'. But the brain is much more material as one can see it through MRI techniques which produce images of it. Or you can also see in the event of an accident, where someone might spill their brains on the road. But as Bhaskar has shown, the brain is not only the organ located inside the skull with which it is most commonly identified, but it extends its influence throughout the body through various intricate neural and other systems. The body receives, processes and responds to information and stimuli and sometimes even to these strange things called thoughts and other cognitive products and even feelings. It can make the heart go faster and then interpret that accelerating heartbeat as a sign of being attracted to someone or to a thought that would say, 'Hey! I am attracted to that person'. So it can start by interpreting its own body and sometimes it misinterprets as well. So, these thoughts can be encoded in language and actions that can be transmitted to other organisms of the same or other species – as Bhaskar pointed out – to be decoded and interpreted further.

The extended brain: Implications for the future

Dr Anurag Mishra: Going back a little bit, we are conceived when a thought, an impulse, an intent and an act meet, when an egg and a sperm fuse together. From which, soon a baby develops out of the fused genetic code and becomes a child and acquires intelligence and capacities in turn to produce information and thoughts; and do things in the world in terms of speech, writing and action and carrying on the paintings and carvings on the walls of the world. Now I want to look at it this way: maybe it can be said that our actions and thoughts were precoded in our genes, as our brains came from our genes and those genes came from our parents and one can trace the evolutionary journey, so on and so forth. If we take a short break from this evolutionary journey and reflect on the present times of the pandemic and realise that our body is full of various other organisms – like bacteria and viruses and in the worst scenario some multicellular parasites – that live inside us. We realise that our DNAs were made up of our ancestors who were in a temporal sense also these bacteria and organisms. However, it is not only this but the realisation that every living being is made up of the same stuff that we are made up of and are in a kind of an inter-communication with each other – even the so-called non-living things like rocks and gases were once living things. And through all these long temporal connections, it becomes all the more interesting to ask, 'Where is our brain?' as Bhaskar pre-empted my question. And, can there ever be 'a' brain? I suspect, as he rightly pointed out, not for very long! It is always 'our' brains, which tends to be widely distributed like the new technology called 'block-chain technology' which I do not claim to understand; and we increasingly share our thoughts through electronic media which, if I may say so, are extensions of our brains. My brain is as equally located in my mobile phone and laptop through which I am connected to this conversation and you all, as it is in my skull; and through that it is connected with every other brain and being in our world.

Any virus whether it is RNA, DNA or any piece of misinformation or disinformation in the electronic format can enter our interconnected brains and cause an attack on our network; similar thing happens with virus attacks on computers, a pattern is produced. It is a fallacy to think of human beings as completely separated from others in terms of either species, nations, religions or academic disciplines. Each identity has administrative uses but to see each identity as a separate entity is a fallacy. The commonality between human and animal, living and non-living, human and artificial intelligence are far greater than the difference, which we ignore at our own peril.

I also think there is only one brain but this one is a little different from Bhaskar's megastructure or apex predator. I think, there is only one brain and that is the Earth. We are speaking, eating, talking and sometimes destroying sprouts of it, and it is our responsibility to extend our intellect to the entire planet and not see our brain as imprisoned in our skulls but rather see that our skull is like a helmet for its protection, not a prison. Likewise is the case with our identities, which are not a trap as they give us some shape and sense to navigate life as a tool, but they shouldn't be our prisons or destinies.

After this long detour, what I want to ask is what are the implications of this conceptualisation of the brain? I believe the implications are first for theory. If we look at the brain in the ways you (Anup) and Bhaskar have talked about, then we have to study anatomy, physiology, pathology and a host of other things about the brain, both differently and again; as well as against what has been thought traditionally. In that sense, both diagnosis and prognosis will have implications. This leads to the important implications that are going to be for practice. What will happen to practice if we locate the brain as situated both inside our skull and outside our body, outside in the social and the cultural, as well as in the neurobiological and genetic milieu? What is beginning to happen is a shift in the way in which we see a person, the way in which we approach a patient and the way we take a case history. As we now ask questions pertaining to a whole host of things like family history of neuronal, physiological and other kinds of diseases, we ask questions pertaining to cultural, social and caste backgrounds. Implications are also there for diagnostic tests as prescribed by say Bhaskar – he will prescribe very different tests, for example, genetic or immunological tests, which in turn would reveal very different things as compared to traditional tests. And all of this comes down directly to treatment. If we take your approaches and treat somebody whether as a psychoanalyst or a psychiatrist or whatever you want to call yourself, the treatment becomes very different.

In that sense, we are engaged here in doing something not only disruptive and integrative but something explosive, because what we are doing now is that we are exploding traditional disciplines and analysis. But how? By first exploding disciplinary boundaries in the sense of 'what you need to know'; we are exploding identitarian boundaries in the sense of 'who all do you need to be this person'; we are also exploding the boundaries of psychiatric, psychotherapeutic and psychoanalytic practice in the sense 'what all do you need to do'. So, in a sense, at the risk of sounding grandiose, what we are doing through this conversation right now is a rather dangerous thing because as we are speaking, we are changing the extant contours of these disciplines. So, this is what I think you two gentlemen are doing. This is what LIILR intends to do through its courses.

Acknowledgement: The authors of this chapter/trialogue would like to thank Shivam Sagar, Junior Fellow in Action Research at Livonics Institute of Integrated Learning and Research (www.liilr.livonics.com/team), for editorial support.

Debt Resources

Chalmers, D. (1996). *The conscious mind*. Oxford University Press.

Damasio, A. (2010). *The self comes to mind*. Pantheon.

Freud, S. (1953). Project for a scientific psychology. In *Standard edition of the complete psychological works of Sigmund Freud* (Vol. 1, pp. 281–397). Hogarth Press. (Original work published 1895)

Freud, S. (1957). The unconscious. In *Standard edition of the complete psychological works of Sigmund Freud* (Vol. 14, pp. 166–204). Hogarth Press. (Original work published 1915)

Johnston, A., & Malabou, C. (2013). *Self and emotional life: Philosophy, psychoanalysis, and neuroscience*. Columbia University Press.

Kandel, E. (1999). Biology and the future of psychoanalysis: A new intellectual framework for psychiatry revisited. *The American Journal of Psychiatry, 156,* 505–524.

Panksepp, J. (1998). *Affective neuroscience: The foundations of human and animal emotions*. Oxford University Press.

Parvizi, J. (2009). Corticocentric myopia: Old bias in new cognitive sciences. *Trends in Cognitive Sciences, 13*(8), 354–359.

Salas, C., Turnbull, O., & Solms, M. (2021). *Clinical studies in neuropsychoanalysis revisited*. Routledge.

Solms, M. (2021). *The hidden spring: A journey to the source of consciousness*. W. W. Norton.

Solms, M., & Panksepp, J. (2012). The 'Id' knows more than the 'ego' admits: Neuropsychoanalytic and primal consciousness perspectives on the interface between affective and cognitive neuroscience. *Brain Sciences, 2*(2), 147–175.

Index

"This book was written by a clinician who is, at the same time, a historian of psychoanalysis and one of the most brilliant thinkers in political psychoanalytic thought. Its chapters, which draw from broad and rich worlds of thought and culture, bear the stamp of the unique historical moment they were written alongside the stamp of generations of psychoanalytic thinking: the immediacy and freshness of free associations alongside uncompromising theoretical and clinical rigor.

This is the literary journey of a writer who is, first and foremost, a reader. Therefore, his writing is always a fascinating correspondence, both with the generations that preceded him and with the generations to come. I can't think of a more crucial or enjoyable book through which one can truly recognize the value of psychoanalysis."

Dana Amir, PhD, *training and supervising analyst, Israel Psychoanalytic Society; professor, head of the interdisciplinary doctoral program in psychoanalysis, Haifa University; author,* Psychoanalysis as Radical Hospitality *(Routledge, 2024)*

"Eran Rolnik builds upon his previous creative and innovative writings and sustains his unique voice and perspective in this new – searching and visionary – work."

Christopher Bollas, PhD, *psychoanalyst and former professor of English; author,* Meaning and Melancholia *(Routledge, 2018)*

"I have been familiar with Eran Rolnik's important contributions to psychoanalysis since reading his 2008 paper about Paula Heimann's analysis. In addition to this early writing, Rolnik treats the reader to his impressive breadth of knowledge that includes his wonderful 2012 book, *Freud in Zion: Psychoanalysis and the Making of Modern Jewish Identity*. His new book, *Psychoanalytic Objects Near and Far:Talking Cure* introduces the reader to Rolnik's skills as a practicing psychoanalyst, teacher, historian, and creative clinician and to his skillful analytic treatment. This is an engaging work that analytic clinicians and thinkers will surely find fascinating and relevant to current analytic thinking."

Lawrence J. Brown, PhD, *training and supervising psychoanalyst, Boston Psychoanalytic Institute; author,* Transformational Processes in Clinical Psychoanalysis *(Routledge, 2018)*

Praise for the German Edition

"Every psychoanalyst, in the course of his clinical experience, develops his own theory of treatment. One seldom encounters a book which portrays the practicing analysts' clinical experience as vividly and masterfully as this book by Eran Rolnik. While reading, one is drawn into Rolnik's analytical treatment room and the way he deals with his patients' problems. We are invited to trace his use of concepts and theories and find ourselves caught up in an internal dialogue with the author, which stimulates us to reflect and further develop our own analytic practice. An extraordinary book!"

Werner Bohleber, PhD, *training and supervising analyst, German Psychoanalytic Association; former editor* PSYCHE; *author,* Destructiveness, Intersubjectivity and Trauma *(Routledge, 2010)*

For Product Safety Concerns and Information please contact our EU
representative GPSR@taylorandfrancis.com
Taylor & Francis Verlag GmbH, Kaufingerstraße 24, 80331 München, Germany